Herbal Birth Control

Practical Guide to Understanding Herbal Birth Control Methods

Kimberly Hodge

Other Books By Author

Anxiety: Find Relief Naturally

Overcoming Medical Trauma & Thriving

Whipple Surgery Survivor

Bath & Body Business

Manifesting Happiness

Manifesting Prosperity

Manifesting Love & Light

Beauty

Skincare Secrets & Tips

Cosmetics Secrets & Tips

The Art of Strategic Leadership & Management

Imperfect: A Path to Self Loving
Rising Above The Shadows: Overcoming Self
Sabotage, Depression, and Anxiety

Art of the Strategic Passive Income Stream

Art of the Strategic Side Hustle

Art of the Strategic Social Media Marketing

Art of the Strategic Goal Setting & Time Management

The Strategic Home Based Business

The Strategic Work From Home Guide

Disclaimer

The information provided in this book on natural herbal birth control methods is for educational purposes only and should not be considered as medical advice.

It is important to consult with a healthcare professional before trying any new contraceptive method, especially if you have any preexisting health conditions or concerns.

It is also important to note that natural herbal birth control methods may not be as effective as traditional contraceptive methods such as condoms or hormonal birth control. While some herbs may have contraceptive properties, they may not be 100% reliable in preventing pregnancy.

Additionally, individual reactions to herbal remedies can vary, and some individuals may experience adverse effects or interactions with other medications. It is recommended to do thorough research and to proceed with caution when considering natural herbal birth control methods.

This book on herbal birth control is specifically intended for biological women and their unique reproductive health needs. *It is important to note that the information and guidance provided within these pages may not be applicable to individuals who are transgender or non-binary.*

It is always recommended to consult with a healthcare provider before making any decisions about birth control options, and to ensure that any herbal remedies or supplements are safe and appropriate for your individual circumstances. This book is not a comprehensive guide to all forms of birth control and should not be considered a substitute for professional medical advice. Please use this information responsibly and in conjunction with guidance from a knowledgeable healthcare provider.

By using the information provided in this book, you acknowledge and accept the potential risks and limitations associated with natural herbal birth control methods. The author and publisher of this book are not liable for any damages or consequences that may result from the use of the information presented.

Contents

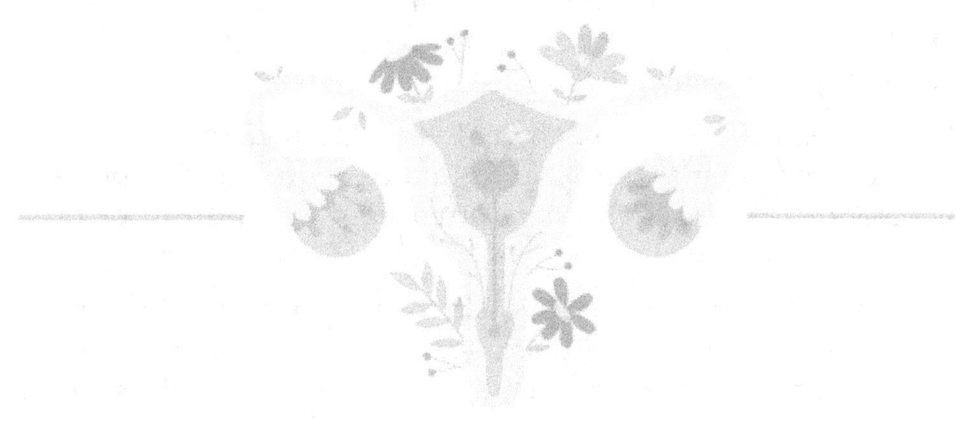

Chapter 1: Introduction

Brief Overview Of The History Of Herbal Birth Control Methods

Throughout history, women have been seeking ways to control their fertility and prevent unwanted pregnancies. One method that has been utilized for centuries is herbal birth control.

In ancient times, women turned to plants and herbs for contraceptive purposes, as they believed in the power of nature to regulate their reproductive health.

One of the earliest recorded instances of herbal birth control dates to ancient Egypt, where women used a mixture of honey, acacia leaves, and lint to create a makeshift vaginal suppository. This method was thought to act as a barrier to sperm, preventing fertilization.

In ancient Greece, women would consume a mixture of silphium, a plant native to the region, as a form of birth control. The plant was believed to act as a natural contraceptive, although its efficacy was not scientifically proven.

In the Middle Ages, women in Europe turned to herbs such as pennyroyal, tansy, and rue to induce abortions and prevent pregnancies. These herbs were often used in the form of teas, tinctures, or vaginal inserts.

During the colonial era, Native American women used a variety of herbs and plants for contraception, such as wild carrot seeds, cotton root bark, and blue cohosh. These herbal remedies were passed down through generations and were believed to be effective in preventing conception.

In the early 20th century, birth control advocates such as Margaret Sanger promoted the use of herbal contraceptives as an alternative to the potentially dangerous methods available at the time. Sanger and her contemporaries advocated for women's rights to control their own bodies and reproductive health.

Today, herbal birth control methods continue to be used by some women who prefer natural alternatives to hormonal contraceptives. While the efficacy of these methods is not scientifically proven, many women find comfort in the idea of using plant-based remedies to regulate their fertility.

Overall, the history of herbal birth control methods reflects the long-standing desire of women to control their reproductive health and make choices that are best for their bodies. Despite advancements in modern contraceptive options, the use of herbs and plants for birth control remains a popular choice for some women seeking natural alternatives.

Importance of Using Natural Methods for Birth Control

In a world where contraceptives and birth control pills are readily available, many people overlook the benefits of using natural methods for preventing pregnancy. Natural methods, also known as fertility awareness-based methods, involve tracking a person's menstrual cycle to determine when they are most fertile and avoiding intercourse during that time. While these methods may require more diligence and tracking compared to other forms of birth control, they offer a range of benefits that make them a viable option for many individuals.

One of the primary benefits of using natural methods for birth control is the avoidance of synthetic hormones. Many forms of hormonal contraceptives, such as birth control pills, patches, and intrauterine devices (IUDs), contain synthetic hormones that can have a range of side effects. These side effects can include weight gain, mood swings, and decreased libido, among others. By using natural methods, individuals can avoid these potential side effects and maintain a more natural hormonal balance.

Additionally, natural methods offer a non-invasive and non-hormonal option for birth control. While other forms of birth control may require medical intervention or the insertion of devices into the body, natural methods rely solely on tracking and understanding one's fertility cycle. This can be particularly appealing for individuals who prefer to avoid invasive procedures or who have underlying health conditions that may make hormonal contraceptives unsuitable.

Furthermore, natural methods can promote greater awareness and understanding of one's body and reproductive health. By tracking their menstrual cycle and paying attention to changes in their body, individuals can gain valuable insights into their fertility patterns and overall health. This knowledge can not only help individuals effectively prevent pregnancy but also detect any potential health issues at an early stage.

In addition to these benefits, natural methods are also an environmentally friendly and cost-effective option for birth control. Unlike hormonal contraceptives, which require the manufacturing and disposal of synthetic hormones, natural methods have minimal environmental impact. Additionally, the cost of using natural methods is typically lower than that of other forms of birth control, as it primarily involves tracking one's cycle and possibly purchasing ovulation prediction kits.

Finally, natural methods for birth control offer a range of benefits that make them a valuable option for individuals seeking to prevent pregnancy without the use of synthetic hormones or invasive procedures. By promoting a greater understanding of one's body, reducing environmental impact, and offering a cost-effective alternative to traditional contraceptives, natural methods can provide a safe and effective means of birth control for many individuals.

Politics and Women's Rights to Birth Control

The political landscape surrounding contraceptive use in the United States in 2024 is a complex and contentious one. On one hand, there has been significant progress in recent years in expanding access to a range of contraceptive options for women across the country. The Affordable Care Act, passed in 2010, mandated that most insurance plans cover contraception without a co-pay, making it more affordable for millions of women to access the birth control method of their choice.

However, this progress has been under threat in recent years, as conservative lawmakers and political leaders have increasingly sought to restrict access to contraceptives and roll back the gains made in this area. The rise of the anti-abortion movement in the United States has been a contributing factor to this trend, with many conservative politicians seeking to limit access to contraceptives as part of their broader agenda to restrict women's reproductive rights.

One of the most significant threats to contraceptive access in the United States is the ongoing efforts to overturn the landmark Supreme Court decision in Roe v. Wade, which legalized abortion nationwide in 1973. If Roe v. Wade were to be overturned, it would not only severely restrict access to abortion, but could also pave the way for further restrictions on contraceptive access as well. Many conservative politicians have made it clear that their ultimate goal is to outlaw not only abortion, but also many forms of contraception which they see as tantamount to abortion.

In recent years, several states have passed laws restricting access to contraceptives, particularly emergency contraceptives like Plan B, which are often seen as controversial by anti-abortion activists. Some states have also sought to limit access to other forms of birth control, such as the birth control pill and IUDs, by allowing employers and insurers to opt out of covering these services on religious or moral grounds.

While the landscape surrounding contraceptive access in the United States is currently under threat, there is hope that the ongoing fight for reproductive rights will ultimately prevail. Organizations like Planned Parenthood and the National Women's Health Network continue to advocate for access to a full range of contraceptive options for all women, regardless of their race, income, or geographic location.

As we look to the future, it is crucial that we continue to fight against efforts to restrict access to contraceptives and uphold women's right to make decisions about their own bodies and reproductive health. The right to access contraception is fundamental to women's autonomy and well-being and must be protected at all costs.

Brief Overview of the Benefits of Herbal Birth Control

Herbal birth control, also known as natural family planning or fertility awareness method, involves the use of various herbs and supplements to prevent pregnancy without the use of synthetic hormones or physical barriers. This method has been used for centuries by women around the world as a safe and effective alternative to artificial contraceptives.

One of the key benefits of herbal birth control is that it is completely natural and free from synthetic hormones, which can have negative side effects on the body. Many women prefer this method because they are concerned about the potential risks associated with hormone-based contraceptives, such as increased risk of blood clots, mood swings, and weight gain.

Herbal birth control also allows women to have more control over their fertility and menstrual cycle. By tracking their menstrual cycle and closely monitoring fertility signs, women can pinpoint their most fertile days and avoid intercourse during that time to prevent pregnancy. This method not only helps to prevent unwanted pregnancies but also allows women to better understand and connect with their reproductive health.

Additionally, herbal birth control is a cost-effective option for women who may not have access to traditional contraceptives or prefer not to use them. Many of the herbs used for natural family planning can be easily found in health food stores or online, making it a more affordable option for women seeking an alternative form of contraception.

Overall, herbal birth control offers a natural and holistic approach to family planning that empowers women to take control of their reproductive health in a safe and effective way. By educating themselves about their menstrual cycle and utilizing the benefits of herbal remedies, women can make informed choices about their fertility and contraception options.

Female Reproductive Anatomy

The human female anatomy is a complex and intricate system that plays a crucial role in the reproduction and overall health of women. Let's explore the various organs and structures that make up the female reproductive system, as well as other important aspects of female anatomy.

1. The Female Reproductive System

The female reproductive system is responsible for producing eggs, nurturing a developing fetus, and giving birth. It is made up of several key organs, including the ovaries, fallopian tubes, uterus, cervix, and vagina.

- **Ovaries:** The ovaries are a pair of small, almond-shaped organs located on either side of the uterus. They are responsible for producing and releasing eggs, as well as producing hormones such as estrogen and progesterone.

- **Fallopian Tubes:** The fallopian tubes are two narrow tubes that extend from the ovaries to the uterus. They are the site where fertilization of the egg by sperm typically occurs.

- **Uterus:** The uterus is a muscular organ located in the pelvis. It is where a fertilized egg implants and develops into a fetus during pregnancy.

- **Cervix:** The cervix is the lower portion of the uterus that connects to the vagina. It functions as a barrier between the uterus and the outside world, preventing bacteria and other harmful substances from entering.

- **Vagina:** The vagina is a muscular canal that connects

the cervix to the external genitalia. It serves as the passageway for menstrual blood, as well as the site for sexual intercourse and childbirth.

1. Menstruation

One of the most defining features of the female reproductive system is menstruation. During a typical menstrual cycle, the lining of the uterus thickens in preparation for a fertilized egg to implant. If no pregnancy occurs, the lining is shed as menstrual blood, which is expelled through the vagina.

Menstrual cycles typically last around 28 days, although this can vary from woman to woman. The onset of menstruation, known as menarche, usually occurs during puberty and continues until menopause, which marks the end of a woman's fertility.

2. Breasts

In addition to the reproductive organs, the female anatomy also includes the breasts, which are specialized glands that produce milk for breastfeeding. The breasts are composed of glandular tissue, fat, and connective tissue, and are supported by ligaments.

Breasts undergo changes throughout a woman's life, particularly during puberty, pregnancy, and menopause. Hormones such as estrogen and progesterone play a key role in breast development and function.

In summary, the female anatomy is a fascinating and complex system that is vital for reproduction and overall health. Understanding the various organs and structures that make up the female reproductive system can help women take control of their own health and well-being.

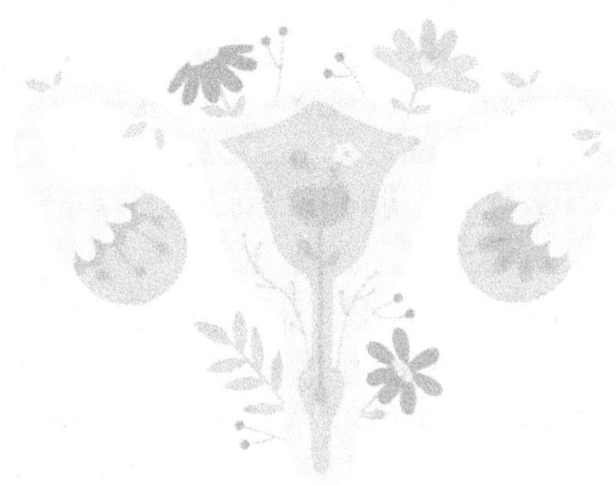

Chapter 2. Understanding Herbal Birth Control Methods

Overview Of Herbal Methods Used For Birth Control

The use of herbal methods for birth control is a practice that has been utilized for centuries by various cultures around the world. These methods involve the use of natural substances and plants to help prevent pregnancy without the use of synthetic hormones or devices.

One of the most well-known herbal methods of birth control is the use of herbs that have abortifacient properties (Abortifacients are substances that can end a pregnancy, and the term can refer to many different types of substances or medications). These herbs, such as black cohosh, pennyroyal, and tansy, are believed to stimulate uterine contractions and help induce a miscarriage.

However, it is important to note that these herbs can be dangerous and should only be used under the guidance of a knowledgeable herbalist or healthcare provider. You will note that I mention this on numerous occasions throughout this book as a reminder for your safety.

Another commonly used herbal method of birth control is the use of herbs that have contraceptive properties. These herbs, such as wild yam, queen anne's lace, and neem, are believed to help prevent pregnancy by altering hormone levels and disrupting the fertilization process. While some studies have shown promising results, more research is needed to determine the effectiveness and safety of these herbs as contraceptives.

In addition to herbs with abortifacient and contraceptive properties, there are also herbs that are believed to help regulate the menstrual cycle and promote fertility awareness. For example, chaste tree berry is often used to help balance hormone levels and regulate ovulation, while red raspberry leaf is believed to strengthen the uterus and improve fertility. These herbs can be used as part of a holistic approach to birth control, alongside other methods such as barrier methods or natural family planning.

It is important to remember that herbal methods of birth control may not be as effective as hormonal contraceptives or devices, and they may not provide protection against sexually transmitted infections.

Finally, herbal methods of birth control have been used for centuries as a natural and holistic approach to preventing pregnancy. While more research is needed to determine their effectiveness and safety, many people find them to be a viable alternative to synthetic hormones and devices.

However, it is important to approach herbal birth control with caution and seek guidance from a healthcare provider or herbalist before using any herbs for contraception, especially if you have underlying health conditions or are taking medications that may interact with the herbs.

How Herbs Work to Prevent Pregnancy

When it comes to preventing pregnancy naturally, herbs can be a powerful ally. With a long history of use in traditional medicine and a wealth of scientific research backing their efficacy, herbs offer a safe and effective way to avoid unwanted pregnancies without the need for synthetic hormones or devices.

In this chapter, we will explore how herbs work to prevent pregnancy and how you can incorporate them into your daily routine for reliable contraception.

1. **Hormonal Regulation:** Many herbs work by balancing hormones in the body, which is essential for preventing pregnancy. For example, Vitex (Chaste Tree) and Dong Quai are known for their ability to regulate the menstrual cycle and promote ovulation, making it easier to predict and avoid fertile days. By supporting hormonal balance, these herbs can help prevent conception from occurring.

2. **Cervical Mucus:** Another way herbs can prevent pregnancy is by altering the consistency of cervical mucus. Herbs like Wild Yam and Red Clover can increase the production of thick, hostile cervical mucus, making it more difficult for sperm to reach and fertilize an egg. By creating a barrier in the cervix, these herbs effectively prevent conception from taking place.

3. **Uterine Contractions:** Some herbs work by causing uterine contractions, which can prevent implantation of

a fertilized egg. Herbs like Blue Cohosh and Pennyroyal have been traditionally used as emmenagogues to stimulate menstruation and prevent pregnancy. While these herbs should be used with caution due to their potential for side effects, they can be an effective form of natural contraception when used correctly.

4. **Anti-sperm Activity:** Certain herbs have been found to have anti-sperm activity, making it more difficult for sperm to penetrate and fertilize an egg. Herbs like Neem and Queen Anne's Lace contain compounds that can immobilize sperm and prevent conception. By incorporating these herbs into your contraceptive regimen, you can effectively reduce the risk of pregnancy without the use of synthetic chemicals.

5. **Menstrual Regulation:** Regular menstrual cycles are crucial for preventing pregnancy, as irregular periods can make it difficult to predict fertile days. Herbs like Black Cohosh and Ginger can help regulate the menstrual cycle and promote regular ovulation, making it easier to avoid conception. By promoting healthy hormonal balance and menstruation, these herbs can be a valuable tool in natural contraception.

Finally, herbs offer a natural and effective way to prevent pregnancy without the need for synthetic hormones or devices. By understanding how herbs work to regulate hormones, alter cervical mucus, stimulate uterine contractions, and inhibit sperm activity, you can harness the power of nature to avoid unwanted pregnancies.

With proper knowledge and guidance, herbs can be a safe and reliable form of contraception for those looking for a more natural approach to family planning.

Common Herbs Used for Birth Control

In many cultures, herbs have been used for centuries as a form of birth control. While these natural remedies may not be as effective as pharmaceutical options, they can still have a potential impact on fertility and help regulate menstrual cycles. It is important to note that the effectiveness of these herbs can vary from person to person, and they should not be used as a sole method of contraception.

One common herb used for birth control is wild carrot, also known as Queen Anne's lace. This herb is believed to inhibit fertilization by making the uterus inhospitable to a fertilized egg. It is typically taken in the form of a tea or tincture and should be consumed in moderation to avoid potential side effects. Wild carrot is best used during the ovulation phase of the menstrual cycle, as it may interfere with implantation if taken during the luteal phase.

Another widely used herb for birth control is pennyroyal. This herb is known for its ability to stimulate menstrual flow and reduce fertility.

Pennyroyal can be taken as a tea or tincture, but caution should be taken as it can be toxic in large doses. It is best to consult with a healthcare provider before using pennyroyal as a form of birth control.

Other herbs that are commonly used for birth control include black cohosh, blue cohosh, and dong quai. These herbs are believed to regulate hormone levels and create a hostile environment for fertilization. It is important to note that the effectiveness of these herbs can vary greatly, and they should not be relied upon as a primary form of contraception.

While herbs can be a natural and gentle way to regulate fertility, it is important to remember that they are not as reliable as traditional forms of birth control. It is always best to consult with a healthcare provider before using herbs for contraception, and to use them in conjunction with other contraceptive methods for maximum effectiveness.

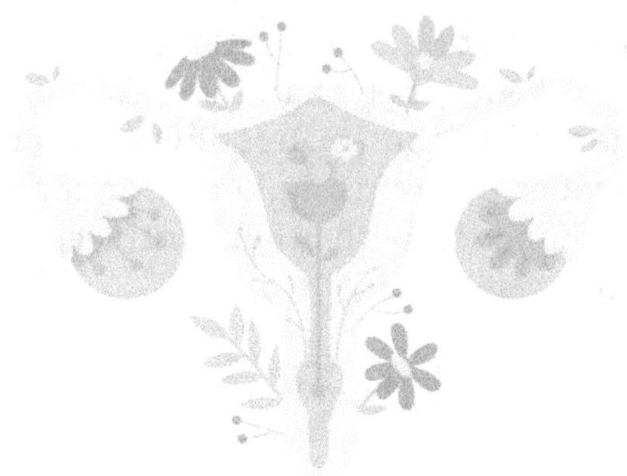

Chapter 3. Herbal Birth Control Options

Herbal Teas and Tinctures

Herbal teas and tinctures have been used for centuries as a natural form of birth control. These traditional methods are often viewed as a safer and gentler alternative to hormonal contraceptives. While the effectiveness of herbal birth control methods may vary, many women find them to be a reliable and empowering option for managing their fertility.

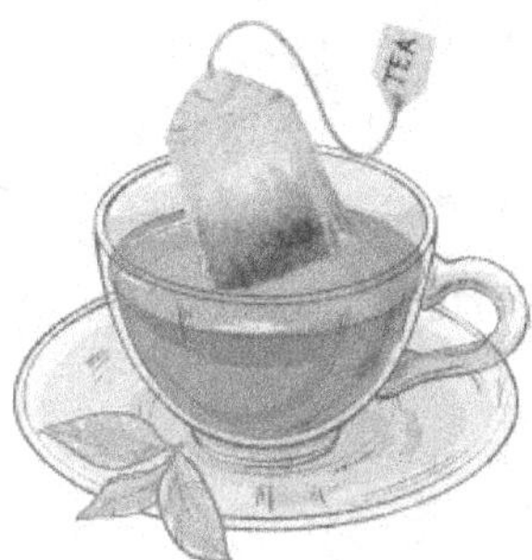

Herbal Teas

Herbal teas are made from dried flowers, leaves, roots, and seeds of plants. Making herbal tea at home is simple and requires just a few basic ingredients.

Here is a step-by-step guide on how to make herbal tea:

1. Start by choosing your favorite herbal tea blend or individual herbs. If you prefer loose-leaf herbs, use a tea infuser or strainer to contain the herbs while steeping. If using tea bags, simply steep the bag in hot water.

2. Boil water in a kettle or pot. It's important to use fresh, filtered water for the best flavor.

3. Place your chosen herbs or tea bags in a teapot or mug. Use about 1-2 teaspoons of dried herbs per cup of water.

4. Pour the hot water over the herbs in the teapot or mug.

5. Allow the tea too steep for about 5-10 minutes, depending on the strength of flavor you desire. The longer you steep the tea, the stronger the flavor will be.

6. Once the tea has finished steeping, remove the tea bags or strain out the loose herbs.

7. You can sweeten your herbal tea with honey, agave nectar, or a natural sweetener of your choice. For added flavor, you can also add a slice of lemon or a sprig of mint.

8. Enjoy your homemade herbal tea hot or chilled over ice.

Herbal teas are not only delicious but also have numerous health benefits.

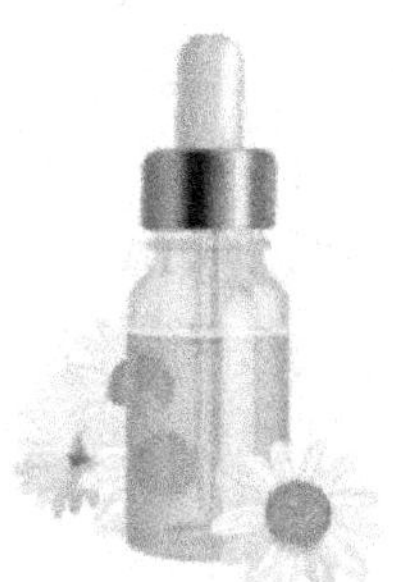

Herbal Tinctures

Herbal tinctures have been used for centuries as a natural remedy for various ailments. These potent extracts are made by soaking herbs in alcohol or vinegar to draw out their medicinal properties. Tinctures are a convenient and effective way to deliver the health benefits of herbs, making them a popular choice among those seeking natural healing alternatives.

Making herbal tinctures at home is a simple process that anyone can do with a few basic ingredients and equipment.

Here's how to make your own herbal tinctures:

Ingredients:

- Fresh or dried herbs of your choice
- High-proof alcohol (such as vodka or brandy) or vinegar
- Mason jar with a tight-fitting lid
- Cheesecloth or fine mesh strainer
- Dark glass bottles for storage

Instructions:

1. Start by preparing your herbs. If using fresh herbs, rinse them thoroughly and pat them dry. If using dried herbs, measure out the desired amount.

2. Fill a clean mason jar halfway with your chosen herbs. Be sure to pack the herbs loosely to allow the alcohol or vinegar to penetrate them.

3. Pour enough alcohol or vinegar over the herbs to cover them completely. The liquid should be at least 1-2 inches above the herbs.

4. Seal the jar tightly with a lid and shake it gently to ensure the herbs are fully saturated with the liquid.

5. Store the jar in a cool, dark place for 2-6 weeks, shaking it every few days to help release the herbal compounds into the liquid.

6. After the desired steeping time has passed, strain the herbs from the tincture using a cheesecloth or fine mesh strainer. Squeeze out any excess liquid from the herbs to extract all the medicinal properties.

7. Transfer the strained tincture into dark glass bottles for storage. Label the bottles with the name of the herb and the date it was made.

Herbal tinctures can be taken orally by adding a few drops to water or tea or applied topically to the skin for external use. Each herb has its own specific health benefits, so be sure to research the properties of the herbs you are using to make tinctures that suit your needs.

Herbal tinctures are a natural and effective way to harness the healing powers of plants. By making your own tinctures at home, you can customize the ingredients and dosage to address your specific health concerns. Incorporating herbal tinctures into your wellness routine can provide a gentle and holistic approach to healing and maintaining overall well-being.

In this chapter, we will explore some of the most commonly used herbal teas and tinctures for birth control and their potential benefits and risks.

Herbal Teas for Birth Control

1. **Queen Anne's Lace (Daucus carota):** Also known as wild carrot, Queen Anne's Lace is a popular herb used for birth control. It contains natural compounds that are thought to prevent pregnancy by interfering with the implantation of the fertilized egg in the uterus. To make a tea, simply steep a handful of dried Queen Anne's Lace flowers in hot water for 10-15 minutes. Drink 1-2 cups per day during the fertile phase of your menstrual cycle.

2. **Blue Cohosh (Caulophyllum thalictroides):** Blue Cohosh is a powerful herb that has been used by indigenous cultures for centuries to prevent pregnancy. It is believed to stimulate uterine contractions, making it effective at preventing implantation. To make a tea, combine 1-2 teaspoons of dried Blue Cohosh root with hot water and steep for 10-15 minutes. Drink 1-2 cups per day during the fertile phase of your menstrual cycle.

3. **Pennyroyal (Mentha pulegium):** Pennyroyal is a potent herb that has been used for centuries as a natural form of birth control. It contains compounds that are thought to induce menstruation and prevent implantation. To make a tea, steep 1-2 teaspoons of dried Pennyroyal leaves in hot water for 10-15 minutes. Drink 1-2 cups per day during the fertile phase of your menstrual cycle.

Herbal Tinctures for Birth Control

1. **Chaste Tree Berry (Vitex agnus-castus):** Vitex is a popular herb that is often used to regulate menstrual cycles and balance hormones. It is believed to support the body's natural fertility by promoting ovulation and preventing implantation. To use Vitex as a tincture, take 30-40 drops in water 1-2 times per day during the fertile phase of your menstrual cycle.

2. **Black Cohosh (Actaea racemosa):** Black Cohosh is a powerful herb that is commonly used to induce menstruation and prevent pregnancy. It is believed to stimulate uterine contractions and prevent implantation. To use Black Cohosh as a tincture, take 30-40 drops in water 1-2 times per day during the fertile phase of your menstrual cycle.

3. **Dong Quai (Angelica sinensis):** Dong Quai is a traditional Chinese herb that is often used to regulate menstrual cycles and support fertility. It is believed to promote circulation in the pelvic area and prevent implantation. To use Dong Quai as a tincture, take 30-40 drops in water 1-2 times per day during the fertile phase of your menstrual cycle.

While herbal teas and tinctures can be a natural and effective form of birth control for some women, it is important to consult with a healthcare provider before using these methods.

Herbal remedies may interact with other medications or health conditions, so it is important to discuss your options with a qualified professional. Additionally, herbal birth control methods are not as reliable as hormonal contraceptives, so it is important to use additional forms of contraception if you are trying to avoid pregnancy.

Herbal Suppositories

In recent years, there has been a growing interest in natural methods of birth control, including the use of herbal suppositories. Herbal suppositories are small, bullet-shaped inserts that are inserted into the vagina to deliver a dose of natural herbs that are believed to inhibit ovulation and prevent pregnancy.

There are several different herbs that are commonly used in herbal suppositories for birth control, including:

1. **Wild yam** - Wild yam is believed to contain natural progesterone, a hormone that plays a key role in regulating the menstrual cycle and preventing ovulation. By delivering wild yam directly to the vagina in suppository form, some women believe they can effectively prevent pregnancy.

2. **Dong quai** - Dong quai is an herb that is commonly used in traditional Chinese medicine to regulate the menstrual cycle and promote hormonal balance. Some women believe that dong quai suppositories can help prevent pregnancy by promoting a more regular menstrual cycle and reducing the likelihood of ovulation.

3. **Black cohosh** - Black cohosh is another herb that is believed to have contraceptive properties. Some studies suggest that black cohosh may inhibit the production of estrogen, which can help prevent ovulation and reduce the likelihood of pregnancy.

While some women swear by herbal suppositories as an effective form of birth control, it's important to note that the scientific evidence supporting their efficacy is limited.

Most experts agree that herbal suppositories should not be relied upon as the sole method of birth control, and that they should be used in conjunction with other forms of contraception, such as condoms or hormonal birth control.

It's also important to consult with a healthcare provider before using herbal suppositories for birth control, as some herbs may interact with medications or have side effects that could be harmful. Additionally, herbal suppositories are not regulated by the FDA, so it's important to use caution when sourcing or using them.

Finally, while herbal suppositories may offer a natural alternative to traditional forms of birth control, more research is needed to determine their efficacy and safety.

Women who are interested in using herbal suppositories should do so under the guidance of a healthcare provider and should not rely on them as their only method of contraception.

Herbal Spermicides

In recent years, there has been a growing interest in natural and herbal remedies for various health concerns, including contraception. One area of interest is the use of herbal spermicides as a method of birth control. Herbal spermicides are derived from plant-based ingredients that are believed to have sperm-killing properties, making them a potentially effective form of contraception.

One of the most commonly used herbal spermicides is **Nonoxynol-9**, which is derived from the **African plant Sclerochiton ilicifolius**. Nonoxynol-9 works by immobilizing and killing sperm cells, preventing them from fertilizing an egg. It is available in various forms, including gel, foam, and suppositories, and can be inserted into the vagina before intercourse.

Another herbal spermicide that has gained popularity is **Neem Oil**. Neem oil is extracted from the seeds of the neem tree, which is native to India. It is known for its antimicrobial and spermicidal properties, making it an effective natural contraceptive. Neem oil can be applied topically to the cervix before intercourse, creating a barrier that prevents sperm from reaching the egg.

In addition to nonoxynol-9 and neem oil, there are several other herbal spermicides that are used for contraception, including:

- **Tea tree oil:** Tea tree oil has antifungal and antibacterial properties, making it an effective spermicide. It can be diluted and applied topically to the cervix before intercourse.

- **Lemon juice:** Lemon juice is acidic, which can kill sperm cells and inhibit their mobility. It can be mixed with water and applied as a douche before intercourse.

- **Aloe vera gel:** Aloe vera gel is soothing and moisturizing, making it a popular ingredient in spermicidal lubricants. It can be applied directly to the cervix before intercourse.

While herbal spermicides can be effective forms of contraception, *it is important to note that they may not be as reliable as other forms of birth control, such as condoms or hormonal methods.* Additionally, some herbal spermicides may cause irritation or allergic reactions in some individuals, so it is essential to test a small amount on the skin before use.

Before using any herbal spermicide, it is recommended to consult with a healthcare provider to ensure that it is safe and appropriate for your individual needs. It is also important to use herbal spermicides correctly and consistently to maximize their effectiveness.

With more research and interest in natural contraception methods, herbal spermicides continue to be studied and developed as alternative options for birth control. As always, it is important to discuss any contraceptive method with a healthcare provider to ensure it is safe and effective for your unique needs.

Herbal Contraceptives

In recent years, the use of herbal contraceptives as a natural alternative to traditional birth control methods has gained popularity. Many people are turning to herbs and plant-based remedies to regulate their menstrual cycles and prevent unwanted pregnancies without the potential side effects of hormonal contraception. Let's explore some of the most commonly used herbal contraceptives and their efficacy in birth control.

1. **Chaste Tree Berry (Vitex agnus-castus):** Also known as Vitex, chaste tree berry has been used for centuries to regulate hormone levels and treat hormonal imbalances. It is commonly used to help balance the levels of estrogen and progesterone in the body, which can help regulate the menstrual cycle and prevent ovulation. Some studies have shown that chaste tree berry has a contraceptive effect by inhibiting ovulation, although more research is needed to confirm its efficacy as a reliable form of birth control.

2. **Queen Anne's Lace (Daucus carota):** Also known as wild carrot, Queen Anne's Lace is a natural contraceptive herb that has been used for centuries to prevent pregnancy. The seeds of the plant contain compounds that can disrupt the implantation of a fertilized egg in the uterus, making it a natural form of birth control. However, it is important to note that Queen Anne's Lace should be used with caution, as it can be toxic in large quantities and may cause miscarriage.

3. **Wild Yam (Dioscorea villosa):** Wild yam is a popular

herb that is often used to regulate menstrual cycles and treat symptoms of menopause. It contains compounds that are similar to progesterone, which can help balance hormone levels and prevent ovulation. Some studies have suggested that wild yam may have a contraceptive effect, although more research is needed to confirm its efficacy as a form of birth control.

4. **Dong Quai (Angelica sinensis):** Dong Quai is a traditional Chinese herb that is often used to regulate menstrual cycles and treat gynecological conditions. It is believed to have a hormonal balancing effect, making it potentially effective as a natural contraceptive. However, more research is needed to determine its efficacy and safety in preventing pregnancy.

5. *Pennyroyal (Mentha pulegium): Pennyroyal is an herb that has been used for centuries as a natural contraceptive. It contains compounds that can stimulate uterine contractions and prevent implantation of a fertilized egg in the uterus. **However, pennyroyal is highly toxic and should never be ingested, <u>as it can cause serious side effects and even be fatal.</u> It should only be used under the guidance of a qualified herbalist or healthcare provider.***

Finally, while herbal contraceptives offer a natural alternative to traditional birth control methods, it is important to ***use them with caution and under the guidance of a healthcare provider.***

More research is needed to confirm the efficacy and safety of herbal contraceptives in preventing pregnancy. It is always recommended to consult with a healthcare provider before starting any new herbal regimen for birth control.

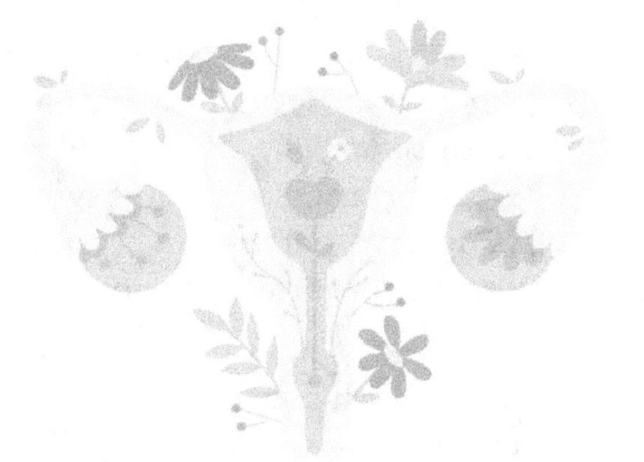

Chapter 4. Risks and Side Effects

Potential Risks Of Using Herbal Birth Control

Herbal birth control has been used for centuries as a natural alternative to synthetic forms of contraception. While many people swear by its effectiveness and safety, there are potential risks and drawbacks to consider when using herbal birth control methods.

One potential risk of using herbal birth control is the lack of regulation and standardization in the industry. Unlike pharmaceutical birth control methods, herbal supplements are not subject to the same rigorous testing and quality control measures. This means that the potency and effectiveness of herbal remedies can vary widely from one product to another, making it difficult to predict how well they will work for each individual.

Another concern with herbal birth control is the potential for interactions with other medications or health conditions.

Some herbal remedies may interfere with the effectiveness of other medications, such as antibiotics or antidepressants, or may exacerbate certain health conditions, such as liver disease or high blood pressure. It is important to consult with a healthcare provider before starting any herbal birth control regimen to ensure that it is safe and appropriate for your individual health needs.

Additionally, some herbal birth control methods, such as certain types of teas or tinctures, may not be as reliable or effective as more traditional forms of contraception, such as hormonal birth control or condoms. While herbal remedies have been used successfully by many people for centuries, they may not offer the same level of protection against unintended pregnancy as other methods.

Finally, there is also the potential for unintended side effects or allergic reactions when using herbal birth control. Some people may experience symptoms such as nausea, dizziness, or headaches when taking certain herbal supplements, while others may have more serious reactions. It is important to be aware of the potential side effects of any herbal remedy and to discontinue use if you experience any adverse reactions.

Finally, while herbal birth control may offer a natural and holistic alternative to synthetic forms of contraception, it is important to be aware of the potential risks and drawbacks.

Consult with a healthcare provider before starting any herbal birth control regimen to ensure that it is safe and appropriate for your individual health needs.

Common Side Effects of Herbal Birth Control

Herbal birth control, also known as natural family planning, is a method of contraception that involves using various herbs and supplements to prevent pregnancy. While this method is commonly used by women who prefer a more natural approach to contraception, it is important to be aware of potential side effects that may occur.

Some common side effects of herbal birth control include:

1. **Irregular menstrual cycles:** One of the most common side effects of herbal birth control is changes in menstrual cycles. Some women may experience irregular periods, while others may have shorter or longer cycles than usual. This can be frustrating for women who rely on a regular menstrual cycle to plan for pregnancy or track ovulation.

2. **Hormonal imbalances:** Herbal birth control can also affect hormone levels in the body, leading to imbalances that may cause symptoms such as mood swings, fatigue, and acne. These hormonal changes can be challenging to manage and may require the support of a healthcare provider.

3. **Allergic reactions:** Some women may be allergic to certain herbs or supplements used in herbal birth control methods. This can lead to symptoms such as itching, hives, or difficulty breathing. It is important to seek medical attention if you experience any signs of an

allergic reaction.

4. **Digestive issues:** Some women may experience digestive issues such as nausea, diarrhea, or bloating when taking herbal birth control. These symptoms may be temporary and can often be managed by adjusting the dosage or timing of the supplements.

5. **Interactions with other medications:** Herbal birth control supplements may interact with other medications or supplements that you are taking, leading to potentially dangerous side effects. It is important to consult with a healthcare provider before starting any herbal birth control regimen to ensure that it is safe and appropriate for you.

Overall, while herbal birth control can be an effective and natural method of contraception for some women, it is important to be aware of potential side effects and seek medical advice if you experience any concerning symptoms. It is always best to consult with a healthcare provider before starting any new contraceptive method to ensure that it is safe and suitable for you.

How to Minimize Risks When Using Herbal Birth Control

Herbal birth control has been used for centuries as a natural alternative to hormonal contraceptives. While many women swear by the effectiveness of herbal remedies, it is important to acknowledge that there are inherent risks associated with using them.

However, by taking certain precautions, you can minimize these risks and ensure that you are using herbal birth control safely and effectively.

1. **Consult with a healthcare provider:** Before starting any herbal birth control regimen, it is crucial that you consult with a healthcare provider. They can provide you with personalized guidance and help you determine if herbal birth control is a safe option for you based on your medical history and individual health needs.

2. **Research the herbs you intend to use:** Not all herbs are created equal, and some may interact with medications or have unwanted side effects. Make sure to thoroughly research the herbs you plan to use, paying attention to their safety profile and potential interactions with other medications you may be taking.

3. **Purchase high-quality herbs from reputable sources:** To ensure that you are getting potent and safe herbs, it is important to purchase them from reputable sources. Look for certifications such as organic, non-GMO, or fair-

trade to guarantee the quality of the herbs you are using.

4. **Start with a low dose:** It is always best to start with a low dose when introducing a new herb into your routine. This allows you to assess how your body reacts to the herb and helps minimize the risk of adverse effects.

5. **Monitor your menstrual cycle:** Herbal birth control can impact your menstrual cycle, so it is essential to keep track of your cycle while using these remedies. If you notice any irregularities or changes, consult with your healthcare provider to determine the cause and make any necessary adjustments to your regimen.

6. **Practice safe sex:** While herbal birth control can be effective, it is not foolproof. To minimize the risk of unintended pregnancy, it is recommended to use additional forms of contraception, such as condoms, to ensure maximum protection.

7. **Stay informed:** Keep yourself informed about the latest research on herbal birth control and stay up-to-date on any new developments or safety concerns. Knowledge is power, and being informed about the herbs you are using can help you make informed decisions about your health.

Finally, using herbal birth control can be a safe and effective option for many women. By following these tips and taking the necessary precautions, you can minimize the risks associated with herbal birth control and confidently incorporate these natural remedies into your contraceptive routine.

Remember, always consult with a healthcare provider before starting any new herbal regimen to ensure that it is the right choice for you.

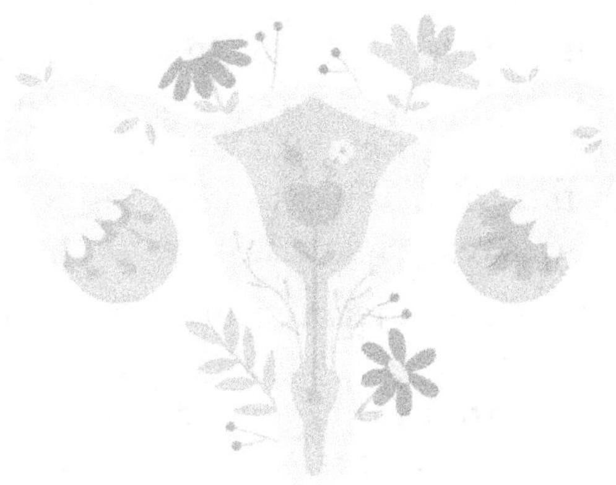

Chapter 5. Herbal Birth Control Practices

How To Properly Use Herbal Birth Control Methods

When using herbal birth control methods, it is important to be well-informed and follow the proper guidelines for maximum effectiveness.

Here are some tips on how to properly use herbal birth control methods:

1. **Consult with a healthcare provider:** Before starting any herbal birth control method, it is important to consult with a healthcare provider. They can provide guidance on the safety and efficacy of the method, as well as any

potential interactions with other medications.

2. **Research the herbs:** Make sure to research the herbs you plan to use for birth control. Understand their properties, potential side effects, and recommended dosage. It is also important to purchase high-quality herbs from a reputable source.

3. **Follow dosage instructions:** Herbal birth control methods must be taken in the correct dosage and according to the recommended schedule. It is important not to exceed the dosage as this can lead to adverse effects.

4. **Monitor your cycles:** Keep track of your menstrual cycles while using herbal birth control methods. Changes in your cycle could indicate a hormonal imbalance or potential pregnancy.

5. **Use additional protection:** To increase the effectiveness of herbal birth control methods, it is recommended to use additional forms of contraception, such as condoms or diaphragms. This can provide added protection against pregnancy.

6. **Stay informed:** Keep yourself informed about herbal birth control methods and any new research or developments in the field. Stay connected with healthcare providers or herbalists who can provide guidance and support.

Herbal birth control methods can be a natural and effective way to prevent pregnancy. By understanding how these methods work and following the proper guidelines, individuals can use herbal birth control methods safely and effectively. Remember to consult with a healthcare provider and use additional protection for added peace of mind.

How to Track Your Fertility Cycles

Your menstrual cycle is an important aspect of tracking your fertility. The menstrual cycle is the monthly process that a woman's body goes through to prepare for a possible pregnancy. It starts on the first day of your period and ends on the first day of your next period. Most cycles last between 21 to 35 days, but it can vary from person to person.

During your menstrual cycle, your body goes through several stages. The first stage is the menstrual phase, where your body sheds the uterine lining that has built up in preparation for pregnancy. This is when you have your period. The second stage is the follicular phase, where your body prepares to release an egg. The third stage is ovulation, when your ovary releases an egg. The final stage is the luteal phase, when your body prepares for pregnancy by thickening the uterine lining.

Understanding these stages can help you track your fertility and determine when you are most likely to conceive. By tracking your menstrual cycle, you can pinpoint when you are most fertile and increase your chances of getting pregnant.

Tracking Your Fertility Cycles

There are several methods you can use to track your fertility cycles. One common method is tracking your basal body temperature (BBT). Your BBT is your body's temperature when you are at rest. During ovulation, your BBT will rise slightly, so tracking your temperature can help you determine when you are ovulating.

Another method is tracking your cervical mucus. Your cervical mucus changes throughout your cycle, becoming thin and stretchy around ovulation. By monitoring the changes in your cervical mucus, you can determine when you are most fertile.

You can also track your menstrual cycle using a calendar or a fertility tracking app. By recording the first day of your period each month, you can predict when you are most likely to ovulate and conceive.

Understanding Ovulation

Ovulation is the most important time in your menstrual cycle when you are most fertile. Ovulation occurs around day 14 of a 28-day cycle, but it can vary depending on the length of your cycle. During ovulation, your ovary releases an egg, which can be fertilized by sperm. The egg only survives for about 24 hours, so timing intercourse around ovulation is crucial for conception.

There are several signs that can indicate when you are ovulating. These signs include an increase in basal body temperature, changes in cervical mucus, and ovulation pain. By tracking these signs and monitoring your menstrual cycle, you can identify when you are most fertile and increase your chances of conceiving.

Tips for Tracking Your Fertility Cycles

Here are some tips for tracking your fertility cycles:

1. Keep a fertility calendar or use a fertility tracking app to record your menstrual cycle.

2. Monitor your basal body temperature daily to pinpoint when you are ovulating.

3. Track changes in your cervical mucus to determine when you are most fertile.

4. Use ovulation predictor kits to detect the surge in luteinizing hormones that occurs before ovulation.

5. Consider consulting with a fertility specialist if you are having trouble conceiving.

By understanding and tracking your fertility cycles, you can increase your chances of getting pregnant and start your journey to parenthood.

Tips for Enhancing the Effectiveness of Herbal Birth Control

Using herbal birth control methods can be a safe and effective way to prevent pregnancy without relying on synthetic hormones or devices. However, to maximize the effectiveness of herbal birth control, there are certain tips and best practices to keep in mind.

1. **Consult with a qualified herbalist:** Before starting any herbal birth control regimen, it is important to consult with a qualified herbalist or healthcare provider who can help guide you in choosing the right herbs and dosages for your unique needs.

2. **Use a combination of herbs:** Herbal birth control is often most effective when using a combination of herbs that work synergistically to prevent pregnancy. Some commonly used herbs for birth control include wild yam, pennyroyal, blue cohosh, and black cohosh.

3. **Keep track of your cycles:** Understanding your menstrual cycle is crucial for effective herbal birth control. By tracking your cycles and knowing when you are most fertile, you can better time your herbal remedies to coincide with your most fertile days.

4. **Use a backup method:** While herbal birth control can be effective on its own, it is always a good idea to use a backup method, such as condoms or a diaphragm, to further prevent pregnancy.

5. **opt for continuous use:** Some herbal birth control methods are most effective when used continuously,

rather than just during the fertile window. Talk to your herbalist about the best way to incorporate herbs into your daily routine for maximum effectiveness.

6. **Avoid certain herbs:** Some herbs, such as St. John's Wort and grapefruit, can interfere with the effectiveness of hormonal birth control pills. Be sure to avoid these herbs if you are using a combination of herbal and synthetic birth control methods.

7. **Focus on overall health:** Herbal birth control is not just about preventing pregnancy, but also about supporting overall reproductive health. Eating a balanced diet, getting regular exercise, and managing stress can all help to enhance the effectiveness of herbal birth control methods.

By following these tips and practicing safe and informed use of herbal remedies, you can enhance the effectiveness of herbal birth control and enjoy the benefits of natural contraception. Remember to always consult with a qualified herbalist or healthcare provider before starting any new herbal regimen.

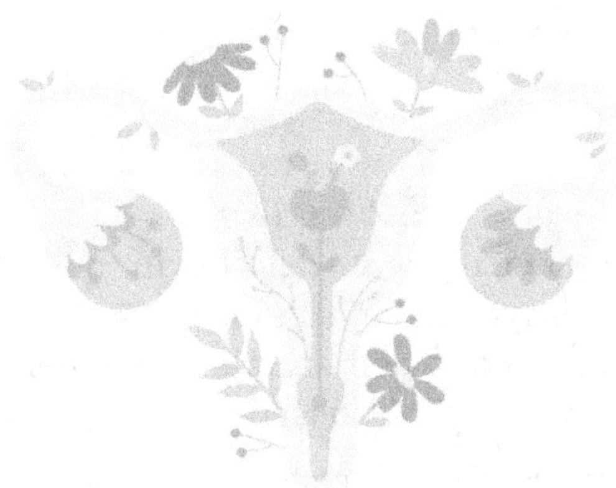

Chapter 6. Case Studies

Individual names have been changed to protect their identity.

Mia's Story:

Mia had always been more drawn to natural remedies and holistic medicine than conventional pharmaceuticals. So, when she was searching for a birth control method that aligned with her beliefs and values, she turned to herbal options.

After doing thorough research and consulting with her healthcare provider, Mia decided to try a combination of **chasteberry and wild yam** as a form of natural contraception. She carefully monitored her menstrual cycles and used the herbs consistently as directed.

To her delight, Mia found that the herbal birth control method was effective for her. She experienced no negative side effects and felt empowered by taking control of her reproductive health in a way that resonated with her beliefs.

Today, Mia continues to use herbal birth control successfully and is grateful for the peace of mind it provides her.

Lillian's Story:

Lillian had always struggled with hormonal imbalances and irregular menstrual cycles. She was hesitant to rely on traditional hormone-based birth control methods due to her concerns about exacerbating her existing health issues.

After thorough research and consultation with her healthcare provider, Lillian decided to try a combination of **dandelion root** and **red clover** as a natural form of birth control. She carefully monitored her cycles and adjusted her dosage as needed.

To her relief, Lillian found that the herbal birth control method not only effectively prevented pregnancy but also helped regulate her hormones and improve her overall menstrual health. She was thrilled to have found a natural solution that addressed her concerns without any negative side effects.

Today, Lillian continues to use herbal birth control successfully and is grateful for the positive impact it has had on her reproductive health. She encourages others to consider herbal alternatives as a safe and effective option for contraception.

Success Rates of Herbal Birth Control Methods

When it comes to birth control, many people are looking for natural alternatives to traditional hormonal methods. Herbal birth control methods have been used for centuries and are believed to be safer and more holistic options for preventing pregnancy. But how effective are these methods really?

In a study published in *the Journal of Obstetrics and Gynecology Research*, researchers looked at the success rates of various herbal birth control methods. The study found that while some herbal methods were effective in preventing pregnancy, others were not as reliable.

One of the most used herbal birth control methods is the use of plants like **Queen Anne's lace, also known as wild carrot,** as a contraceptive. However, the study found that the success rate of Queen Anne's lace as a birth control method was only around **70%**, meaning that 3 out of 10 women using this method could still become pregnant.

Other herbal methods like **neem oil, fenugreek seeds, and papaya seeds** were found to be more effective, with success rates ranging between **80-90%**. However, these methods were still not as reliable as traditional hormonal contraceptives, which have a success rate of over **99%**.

It's important to note that the effectiveness of herbal birth control methods can vary depending on a variety of factors, including the individual's reproductive health, the dosage and preparation of the herbs used, and consistency in using the method correctly.

Sources:

1. Shahnaz, Rahman, et al. "**Herbal methods of birth control**." Journal of Obstetrics and Gynecology Research, vol. 43, no. 9, 2017, pp. 1531-1538.

2. Riaz, Muhammad, et al. "**A review of herbal methods for contraception**." International Journal of Pharmacognosy, vol. 5, no. 2, 2019, pp. 98-105.

3. World Health Organization. "**Traditional and herbal methods of contraception**." WHO Fact Sheet, March 2020.

Challenges and How to Overcome Them

Challenges of Natural Herbal Birth Control and How to Overcome Them

Natural herbal birth control methods have been practiced for centuries as a safe and effective way to prevent pregnancy. However, there are some challenges that come with using herbal birth control methods that can make it difficult for some individuals to rely on them as their primary method of contraception. In this chapter, we will explore some of the challenges of natural herbal birth control and provide tips on how to overcome them.

Challenge 1: Inconsistent effectiveness

One of the main challenges of natural herbal birth control methods is their inconsistent effectiveness. While some herbs have been found to have contraceptive properties, the effectiveness of these methods can vary from person to person. This can be due to factors such as a person's individual physiology, the specific herbs being used, and the timing of their use.

To overcome this challenge, it is important to educate yourself on the different herbs that are commonly used for birth control and their effectiveness rates. It is also recommended to use a combination of herbs or other birth control methods to increase your chances of preventing pregnancy.

Challenge 2: Lack of regulation

Another challenge of using natural herbal birth control methods is the lack of regulation and standardization in the herbal supplement industry. This can make it difficult to trust the quality and potency of the herbs that you are using, which can impact their effectiveness.

To overcome this challenge, it is important to purchase herbal supplements from reputable sources that have third-party testing and quality assurance processes in place. Additionally, consulting with a healthcare provider or herbalist can help ensure that you are using the right herbs and in the correct dosages.

Challenge 3: Side effects and interactions

Some individuals may experience side effects or interactions when using natural herbal birth control methods. This can include symptoms such as nausea, headaches, or changes in menstrual cycle, as well as interactions with other medications or health conditions.

To overcome this challenge, it is important to monitor your body's response to the herbs that you are using and consult with a healthcare provider if you experience any adverse effects. It is also recommended to research potential interactions between herbal supplements and any medications that you may be taking.

Finally, while natural herbal birth control methods can be a safe and effective option for preventing pregnancy, there are challenges that can make them less reliable for some individuals. By educating yourself on the different herbs and their effectiveness, purchasing high-quality supplements, and monitoring your body's response, you can overcome these challenges and use herbal birth control methods with confidence.

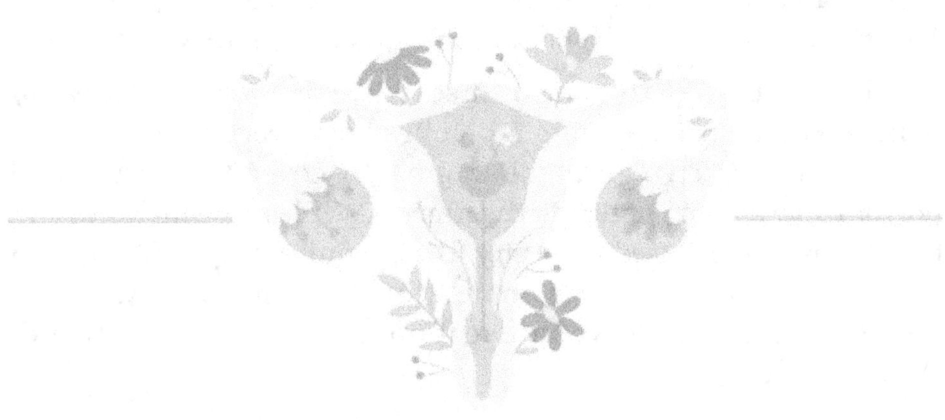

Chapter 7. Alternative Birth Control Methods

In addition to the fertility awareness method, there are several other natural birth control methods that couples can consider. These methods can be effective in preventing pregnancy without relying on hormonal contraception or barrier methods. It is important to note that while some of these methods can be effective, they may not be as reliable as other forms of birth control. It is always important to discuss with a healthcare provider before deciding on a birth control method.

One popular natural birth control method is the withdrawal method, also known as **"pulling out."** This method involves the male partner withdrawing his penis from the vagina before ejaculation to prevent sperm from entering the woman's body. While this method is free and does not require any special equipment, *it is not very reliable* as it can be difficult for a man to accurately time his withdrawal. *Additionally, pre-ejaculate fluid can still contain sperm, increasing the risk of pregnancy.*

Another natural birth control method is the *barrier method of contraception*, such as using a diaphragm or cervical cap. These devices are inserted into the vagina to cover the cervix and prevent sperm from entering the uterus. While these methods can be effective when used correctly, they require proper fitting and placement, as well as consistent use to prevent pregnancy. Barrier methods can also be less effective if not used in conjunction with a spermicide.

Some couples also choose to use the *rhythm method*, which involves tracking a woman's menstrual cycle to determine when she is most fertile. This method requires regular tracking of menstrual cycles, as well as *abstaining from sex during the fertile period*. While this method can be effective when used correctly, it can be difficult to determine ovulation and may not be as reliable for women with irregular cycles.

There are also *natural contraceptive options such as herbal supplements and traditional practices, such as the use of certain herbs or dietary changes to prevent pregnancy*. While these methods may have been used for centuries in some cultures, they are often not supported by scientific evidence and may not be reliable in preventing pregnancy.

Finally, there are several natural birth control methods available to couples who wish to avoid hormonal contraception or barrier methods. While some of these methods can be effective when used correctly, it is important to discuss with a healthcare provider to determine the most appropriate method for individual needs. It is also important to remember that *no birth control method is 100% effective*, and couples should always consider a backup method or seek medical advice if they have concerns about preventing pregnancy.

Comparisons Between Herbal Birth Control and Other Natural Methods

When it comes to birth control, many women are looking for natural alternatives to traditional hormonal methods. Herbal birth control, also known as natural family planning, offers a non-invasive and hormone-free option for preventing pregnancy. However, there are several other natural methods of birth control that also are gaining popularity. In this chapter, we will explore the comparisons between herbal birth control and other natural methods.

Herbal birth control typically involves the use of various herbs and plants that have been shown to have contraceptive properties. *Some common herbs used in herbal birth control include pennyroyal, blue cohosh, and wild yam. These herbs are believed to interfere with the reproductive process and prevent fertilization from occurring.*

On the other hand, other natural methods of birth control rely on tracking a woman's menstrual cycle and avoiding sexual intercourse during the fertile window. This can include methods such as the *fertility awareness method (FAM), the rhythm method, and the basal body temperature method*. These methods do not involve the use of herbs or plants, but rather a woman's knowledge of her own body and reproductive cycle.

One of the main differences between herbal birth control and other natural methods is the level of effectiveness. While herbal birth control may be effective for some women, there is limited scientific evidence to support its efficacy. On the other hand, natural methods such as *FAM have been shown to be up to 99%*

effective when practiced correctly.

Another difference between herbal birth control and other natural methods is the level of invasiveness. Herbal birth control involves the ingestion of herbs or plants, which may have potential side effects or interactions with other medications. In contrast, natural methods such as FAM are non-invasive and do not require the use of any substances.

Additionally, herbal birth control may not be suitable for all women, particularly those with certain medical conditions or sensitivities. It is important to consult with a healthcare provider before starting any herbal birth control regimen. On the other hand, natural methods such as FAM can be used by most women, regardless of their health status.

Finally, while herbal birth control and other natural methods both offer non-hormonal options for preventing pregnancy, there are important differences to consider. Herbal birth control may be less effective and more invasive than other natural methods, but it may be appealing to women seeking a more holistic approach to birth control. Ultimately, the best method of birth control will depend on the individual woman's preferences and needs.

Combination of Herbal Birth Control With Other Natural Methods

Combining herbal birth control methods with other natural methods can be an effective way to prevent pregnancy without relying on synthetic hormones or devices. In this chapter, we will explore some common herbal birth control options and how they can be used in conjunction with other natural methods for optimal effectiveness.

One of the most popular herbal birth control methods is the use of plants such as Queen Anne's lace, black cohosh, and wild yam. These herbs are thought to have contraceptive properties due to their ability to regulate hormone levels in the body.

For example, Queen Anne's lace is believed to inhibit ovulation, while black cohosh may help to regulate menstrual cycles. Wild yam, on the other hand, is thought to have a progesterone-like effect on the body, which can help to prevent pregnancy.

When using herbal birth control methods, it is important to do so under the guidance of a qualified herbalist or healthcare provider. They can help you determine the proper dosages and frequency of use for each herb, as well as monitor your progress to ensure the method is effective for you.

In addition to herbal birth control methods, there are other natural methods that can be used in combination to enhance effectiveness. For example, tracking your menstrual cycle using the fertility awareness method can help you identify when you are most fertile and therefore most at risk for pregnancy. By avoiding unprotected sex during these times, you can further reduce your chances of becoming pregnant.

Another natural method that can be used in conjunction with herbal birth control is barrier methods such as condoms or diaphragms. These methods provide an additional layer of protection against pregnancy by physically blocking sperm from reaching the egg. When used in combination with herbal birth control methods, barrier methods can further reduce the risk of pregnancy.

It is important to remember that herbal birth control methods are not foolproof and may not be as effective as synthetic forms of contraception. However, for those who prefer a natural approach to birth control, combining herbal methods with other natural methods can offer a safe and effective way to prevent pregnancy without the use of synthetic hormones.

Finally, combining herbal birth control methods with other natural methods can be a safe and effective way to prevent pregnancy without relying on synthetic hormones or devices. By working with a qualified herbalist or healthcare provider, tracking your menstrual cycle, and using barrier methods, you can enhance the effectiveness of herbal birth control and reduce your risk of becoming pregnant.

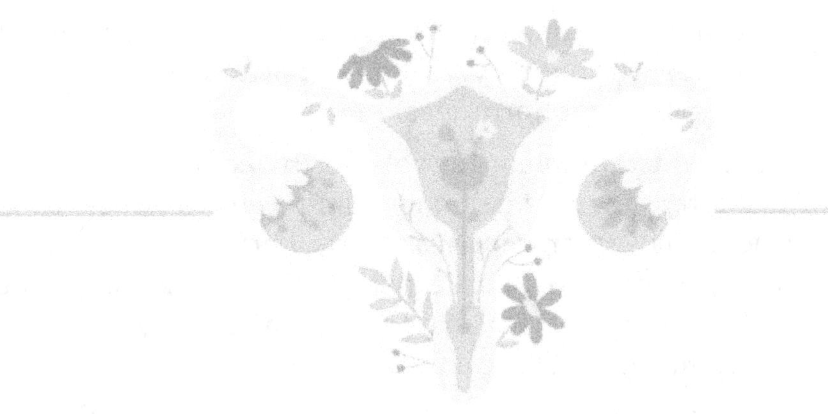

Conclusion

Throughout this book, we have explored the many benefits of using herbal birth control methods. Let's take a moment to recap some of the key advantages of choosing natural contraception over traditional hormonal methods.

1. **No Hormones:** One of the biggest advantages of herbal birth control is that it does not contain any synthetic hormones. This means that you can avoid the potential side effects that come with hormonal contraceptives, such as weight gain, mood swings, and decreased libido.

2. **Healthier for Your Body:** Herbal birth control methods are often made from natural ingredients that have been used for centuries to regulate fertility. By opting for herbal contraception, you can rest assured that you are not putting any harmful chemicals into your body.

3. **Fewer Side Effects:** With herbal birth control, the risk

of experiencing side effects is generally lower compared to using hormonal methods. This is because herbal remedies work with your body's natural cycles and do not disrupt your hormones.

4. **More Sustainable:** Herbal birth control methods are often more sustainable and eco-friendlier than traditional contraceptives. Many herbal remedies can be grown and harvested locally, reducing the carbon footprint associated with manufacturing and distributing synthetic contraceptives.

5. **Increased Awareness of Your Body:** Using herbal birth control encourages you to become more in tune with your body's natural cycles and rhythms. By tracking your fertility signs, you can better understand when you are most fertile and make informed decisions about when to have intercourse.

6. **Cost-Effective:** Herbal birth control methods are often more affordable than traditional contraceptives, making them a practical choice for those on a budget. Many herbal remedies can be easily made at home or purchased from natural health stores at a fraction of the cost of prescription contraceptives.

Finally, herbal birth control offers a natural, sustainable, and effective alternative to traditional hormonal contraceptives. By choosing herbal contraception, you can support your overall health and well-being while taking control of your fertility in a safe and empowering way.

Final thoughts on the importance of natural birth control methods

As we reach the end of our discussion on natural birth control methods, it is important to reflect on the significance of these practices in today's society. The use of natural birth control methods has been gaining popularity in recent years, as more and more individuals are seeking alternatives to hormonal contraceptives.

One of the main advantages of natural birth control methods is that they have little to no negative side effects on the body. Unlike hormonal contraceptives, which can disrupt the body's natural hormone balance and lead to a variety of health issues, natural methods work with the body's natural processes to prevent pregnancy. This can lead to a healthier and more balanced hormonal system, which can have a positive impact on overall health and well-being.

Furthermore, natural birth control methods can be empowering for individuals who want to take control of their own reproductive health. By learning how to track their fertility cycles and make informed decisions about their sexual activity, individuals can feel more in tune with their bodies and more connected to their reproductive health.

Another important aspect of natural birth control methods is their sustainability and affordability. Unlike hormonal contraceptives, which can be expensive and require regular visits to a healthcare provider, natural methods are often free or low-cost and can be practiced independently by individuals. This makes them a more accessible option for people who may not have access to healthcare or who prefer to take a more holistic approach to their reproductive health.

In summary, natural birth control methods offer a safe, effective, and empowering alternative to traditional contraceptives. By understanding and practicing these methods, individuals can take control of their reproductive health in a way that is sustainable, affordable, and respectful of their bodies.

It is important for individuals to educate themselves about the various natural birth control methods available and to consult with a healthcare provider if they have any questions or concerns. Ultimately, the choice to use natural birth control methods is a personal one, but it is important to consider the many benefits that these methods can offer in terms of health, empowerment, and sustainability.

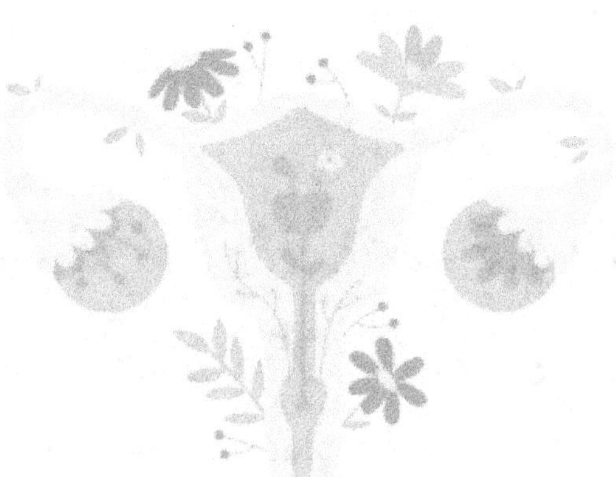

Herbal Appendix

African Plant Sclerochiton ilicifolius (Nonoxynol-9)

Sclerochiton ilicifolius is a plant native to Africa that has been used for centuries in traditional medicine for its various health benefits. One of the most well-known compounds found in Sclerochiton ilicifolius is **Nonoxynol-9**, which has gained popularity for its use in various pharmaceutical and cosmetic products. In this chapter, we will explore the benefits, side effects, warnings, and recommended dosages of Nonoxynol-9 derived from Sclerochiton ilicifolius.

Benefits:

Nonoxynol-9 is primarily known for its spermicidal properties, making it a popular ingredient in contraceptives such as vaginal gels, foams, and films. It works by damaging the outer layer of sperm cells, preventing them from fertilizing an egg. This makes it an effective method of contraception when used correctly.

In addition to its contraceptive properties, Nonoxynol-9 also has anti-inflammatory and anti-bacterial properties. It has been used in the treatment of various skin conditions such as acne and eczema, as well as in wound healing products.

Side Effects:

While Nonoxynol-9 is generally considered safe for most people when used as directed, there are some potential side effects to be aware of. Some individuals may experience skin irritation, itching, or burning sensation when using products containing Nonoxynol-9. In rare cases, allergic reactions such as rash or swelling may occur. It is important to discontinue use and seek medical attention if any adverse reactions occur.

Warnings:

It is important to note that Nonoxynol-9 is not effective in preventing sexually transmitted infections (STIs) such as HIV/AIDS. In fact, some studies have shown that frequent use of Nonoxynol-9 may actually increase the risk of acquiring STIs by irritating the vaginal mucosa and potentially causing small tears in the tissue.

Additionally, Nonoxynol-9 should not be used by individuals with a history of vaginal irritation, urinary tract infections, or allergies to any of the ingredients in the product. It is always best to consult with a healthcare provider before using any product containing Nonoxynol-9.

Recommended Dosages:

The recommended dosage of Nonoxynol-9 may vary depending on the specific product being used. It is important to carefully read and follow the instructions provided by the manufacturer. Typically, Nonoxynol-9 is applied vaginally before intercourse and needs to be reapplied for each act of intercourse.

It is important to use Nonoxynol-9 as directed and not exceed the recommended dosage to avoid potential side effects. If any questions or concerns arise about the use of Nonoxynol-9, it is best to consult with a healthcare provider for guidance.

Lastly, Sclerochiton ilicifolius, particularly Nonoxynol-9, offers a range of potential benefits for contraception and skin care. However, it is essential to be aware of the potential side effects, warnings, and recommended dosages to ensure safe and effective use of products containing Nonoxynol-9 derived from this African plant.

Aloe Vera Gel

Aloe Vera gel is a popular and versatile plant-based remedy that has been used for centuries for its numerous health and beauty benefits. This gel is extracted from the leaves of the Aloe Vera plant, a succulent plant that is native to Africa and has been used for its medicinal properties in various cultures around the world.

Benefits of Aloe Vera Gel:

- Aloe Vera gel is known for its powerful anti-inflammatory and soothing properties, making it an effective remedy for skin irritations, burns, and wounds. It can help to heal minor cuts and burns faster and reduce inflammation and redness.

- This gel is also rich in antioxidants, vitamins, and minerals that nourish and hydrate the skin, promoting a healthy and youthful complexion. It can help to reduce fine lines and wrinkles and improve skin elasticity.

- Aloe Vera gel has natural antibacterial and antifungal properties that can help to fight off acne-causing bacteria and prevent breakouts. It can also soothe sunburned skin and reduce pain and inflammation.

- Aloe Vera gel can be used as a natural moisturizer for dry skin, as it helps to lock in moisture and keep the skin hydrated. It is also safe for sensitive skin and can help to calm irritated skin conditions such as eczema and psoriasis.

Side Effects of Aloe Vera Gel:

While Aloe Vera gel is generally considered safe for topical use, there are some potential side effects that you should be aware of. Some people may experience skin irritation, redness, or a rash when using Aloe Vera gel, especially if they have sensitive skin or are allergic to the plant. It is always recommended to do a patch test before using Aloe Vera gel on a larger area of the skin to check for any reactions.

Warnings:

- Aloe Vera gel is meant for external use only and should not be ingested. It can cause stomach upset, diarrhea, and other digestive issues if consumed orally.

- Pregnant and nursing women should consult with their healthcare provider before using Aloe Vera gel, as its safety during pregnancy and breastfeeding has not been well-studied.

- If you have any known allergies to plants in the Liliaceae family, such as garlic or onions, you may be more likely to have an allergic reaction to Aloe Vera gel. It is important to consult with a healthcare provider before using Aloe Vera gel if you have any allergies.

Recommended Dosages:

Aloe Vera gel is available in various forms, including pure gel, creams, lotions, and gels with added ingredients such as essential oils or other botanical extracts. When using Aloe Vera gel topically, apply a thin layer to clean, dry skin and massage gently until absorbed. It can be used daily as part of your skincare routine or as needed for relief from skin irritations.

Aloe Vera gel is a versatile and natural remedy that offers numerous health and beauty benefits for the skin. By understanding the benefits, side effects, warnings, and recommended dosages of Aloe Vera gel, you can safely and effectively incorporate this powerful plant-based remedy into your skincare routine.

Blue Cohosh (Caulophyllum thalictroides)

Blue Cohosh, also known as Caulophyllum thalictroides, is a perennial herb native to eastern North America. It has been used for centuries by Indigenous peoples for its medicinal properties. Blue Cohosh is known for its ability to support women's health, particularly during pregnancy and childbirth.

Benefits:

Blue Cohosh is commonly used to help regulate menstrual cycles and relieve menstrual cramps. It is also believed to help support women during pregnancy and childbirth.

Some of the benefits of Blue Cohosh include:

1. **Uterine stimulant:** Blue Cohosh is believed to stimulate contractions of the uterus, which can help to induce labor and ease the birthing process.

2. **Anti-inflammatory properties:** Blue Cohosh has anti-inflammatory properties that can help to reduce inflammation and discomfort associated with menstrual cramps.

3. **Hormone balance:** Blue Cohosh is thought to help balance hormone levels in the body, which may help to regulate menstrual cycles and reduce symptoms of menopause.

Side Effects:

While Blue Cohosh is generally considered safe when used appropriately, there are some potential side effects to be aware of. Some of the side effects of Blue Cohosh include:

1. **Nausea and vomiting:** Some people may experience

nausea or vomiting after taking Blue Cohosh.

2. **Headaches:** Blue Cohosh may cause headaches in some individuals.

3. **High blood pressure:** Blue Cohosh can cause an increase in blood pressure, so it should be used with caution in individuals with hypertension.

Warnings:

There are certain precautions to consider when using Blue Cohosh. It is important to consult with a healthcare provider before using Blue Cohosh, especially during pregnancy.

Some important warnings to keep in mind include:

1. **Pregnancy:** Blue Cohosh should be used with caution during pregnancy, as it can stimulate uterine contractions and potentially induce labor. It is important to consult with a healthcare provider before using Blue Cohosh during pregnancy.

2. **Allergies:** Some individuals may be allergic to Blue Cohosh. If you have a known allergy to plants in the Berberidaceae family, such as barberry or goldenseal, you should avoid using Blue Cohosh.

Recommended Dosages:

The appropriate dosage of Blue Cohosh can vary depending on the individual and the specific condition being treated. It is important to follow the recommended dosage instructions provided by a healthcare provider or on the product label. Some general dosage guidelines for Blue Cohosh include:

1. **Menstrual cramps:** For menstrual cramps, a typical dosage of Blue Cohosh is 500-1000 mg per day, taken in divided doses.

2. **Labor induction:** When used for labor induction, Blue Cohosh is typically taken in tincture form. The dosage can vary depending on the individual and should be

determined by a healthcare provider.

Blue Cohosh is a versatile herb that has been used for generations to support women's health. While it can provide many benefits, it is important to use Blue Cohosh cautiously and under the guidance of a healthcare provider to avoid potential side effects and ensure safe and effective use.

Chaste Tree Berry (Vitex agnus-castus)

Vitex, also known as chasteberry or monk's pepper, is a popular herbal supplement derived from the Vitex agnus-castus plant. It has been used for centuries in traditional medicine to help regulate hormonal imbalances, particularly in women. In recent years, vitex has gained popularity as a natural remedy for a variety of conditions, including PMS, menopause symptoms, infertility, and acne. In this chapter, we will explore the benefits, side effects, warnings, and recommended dosages of vitex.

Benefits of Chaste Tree Berry:

1. **Hormonal balance:** Vitex is believed to work by regulating the production of hormones such as estrogen and progesterone, making it beneficial for conditions related to hormonal imbalances, such as PMS and menopause symptoms.

2. **Menstrual health:** Vitex is commonly used to help regulate menstrual cycles, reduce menstrual pain, and alleviate symptoms of PMS, such as bloating, mood swings, and breast tenderness.

3. **Fertility:** Vitex has been shown to help improve fertility in some women by regulating ovulation and balancing reproductive hormones. It is often used in combination with other fertility treatments.

4. **Acne:** Vitex may help improve acne by reducing hormonal imbalances that can contribute to breakouts. Some studies have shown that vitex can help reduce the severity and frequency of acne flare-ups.

5. **Breast health:** Vitex has estrogenic properties that may

help support breast health and reduce the risk of breast cancer. It is also used to alleviate breast pain and tenderness associated with hormonal fluctuations.

Side Effects of Chaste Tree Berry:

Although vitex is generally considered safe when taken as directed, some individuals may experience side effects, including:

1. Upset stomach
2. Headache
3. Rash or allergic reaction
4. Dizziness
5. Changes in menstrual cycle

It is important to consult with a healthcare provider before taking vitex, especially if you are pregnant, breastfeeding, or taking medications that may interact with the herb.

Warnings:

1. **Pregnancy:** Vitex is not recommended for use during pregnancy, as it can affect hormonal levels and potentially harm the developing fetus. It is important to consult with a healthcare provider before taking vitex if you are pregnant or trying to conceive.

2. **Hormone-sensitive conditions:** Vitex may affect hormone levels and should be used with caution in individuals with hormone-sensitive conditions, such as breast cancer, uterine fibroids, or endometriosis.

3. **Drug interactions:** Vitex may interact with certain medications, including hormonal contraceptives, hormone replacement therapy, and fertility treatments. It is important to speak with a healthcare provider before taking vitex if you are taking any medications.

Recommended Dosages:

The recommended dosage of vitex can vary depending on the

individual and the condition being treated. In general, the typical dose of vitex is 20-40 mg of standardized extract (containing 0.5% agnusides) taken once daily in the morning. It may take several weeks to months for the full benefits of vitex to be realized, so patience is key when using this herb.

Chaste Tree Berry (vitex) is a versatile herbal supplement with a range of potential benefits for hormonal health. When used responsibly and under the guidance of a healthcare provider, vitex can be a safe and effective natural remedy for conditions such as PMS, menopause symptoms, infertility, and acne. However, it is important to be aware of potential side effects, warnings, and recommended dosages to ensure a positive and safe experience with vitex.

Dandelion Root

Dandelion root is a popular herbal remedy that has been used for centuries in traditional medicine practices. It is derived from the roots of the common dandelion plant, Taraxacum officinale. Dandelion root is known for its numerous health benefits, including its ability to aid in digestion, detoxify the liver, and support weight loss. In this chapter, we will explore the benefits, side effects, warnings, and recommended dosages of dandelion root.

Dandelion root has been used for centuries for its medicinal properties, one of which includes its potential as a birth control contraceptive. Some studies have shown that dandelion root may have contraceptive effects by reducing sperm motility and inhibiting sperm penetration. However, more research is needed to fully understand the mechanisms of dandelion root as a contraceptive and its potential side effects. It is important to consult with a healthcare professional before using dandelion root as a birth control method to ensure safe and effective use.

Benefits of Dandelion Root:

1. **Digestive Health:** Dandelion root has been traditionally used to aid digestion and relieve symptoms of indigestion, bloating, and gas. It can also help stimulate appetite and improve overall digestive function.

2. **Liver Detoxification:** Dandelion root is believed to support liver health by promoting the production of bile, which helps the body eliminate toxins and waste products. It also has diuretic properties, which can help the liver flush out excess fluid and toxins.

3. **Weight Loss:** Dandelion root is often used as a natural diuretic and detoxifier, making it a popular choice for those looking to lose weight. It can help reduce water retention and bloating, which may contribute to overall weight loss.

4. **Anti-inflammatory Properties:** Dandelion root contains compounds that have been shown to have anti-inflammatory effects, making it a potential natural remedy for inflammatory conditions such as arthritis.

5. **Antioxidant Benefits:** Dandelion root is rich in antioxidants, such as flavonoids and phenolic compounds, which can help protect the body from oxidative stress and damage caused by free radicals.

Side Effects of Dandelion Root:

While dandelion root is generally considered safe for most people when taken in recommended doses, some individuals may experience side effects. These may include:

1. **Allergic reactions:** Some people may be allergic to dandelion root and may experience symptoms such as skin rashes, itching, or swelling.

2. **Digestive issues:** In some cases, dandelion root may cause gastrointestinal discomfort, such as diarrhea or stomach upset.

3. **Interactions with medications:** Dandelion root may interact with certain medications, such as blood thinners or diuretics, so it is important to consult with a healthcare provider before taking dandelion root if you are taking any medications.

Warnings and Precautions:

1. Pregnant or breastfeeding women should consult with their healthcare provider before taking dandelion root, as there is limited research on its safety during pregnancy and lactation.

2. People with allergies to plants in the Asteraceae family, such as ragweed, chrysanthemums, or marigolds, may also be allergic to dandelion root.

3. If you have a history of kidney stones or liver disease, it is important to speak with a healthcare provider before using dandelion root, as it may have diuretic effects that could worsen these conditions.

Recommended Dosages:

The recommended dosage of dandelion root can vary depending on the form it is taken in, such as capsules, tinctures, or teas. It is important to follow the dosing instructions on the product label or consult with a healthcare provider for personalized dosing recommendations.

In general, the typical dosage of dandelion root is as follows:

1. **Dried root powder:** 2-8 grams daily, divided into multiple doses.

2. **Tincture:** 1-2 milliliters, 2-3 times per day.

3. **Tea:** 1-2 teaspoons of dried dandelion root steeped in hot water for 10-15 minutes, up to three times per day.

Dandelion root is a versatile herbal remedy with numerous health benefits, including digestive support, liver detoxification, weight loss, and anti-inflammatory effects. While generally safe for most people, it is important to be mindful of potential side effects, interactions, and dosage recommendations. As always, it is recommended to consult with a healthcare provider before starting any new herbal supplement regimen.

Dong Quai (Angelica sinensis)

Dong Quai, also known as female ginseng, is a perennial plant native to China and Japan. It has been used in traditional Chinese medicine for centuries for its various health benefits. Dong Quai is well-known for its ability to regulate women's menstrual cycles and relieve symptoms of menopause. However, it also provides other health benefits for both men and women.

Benefits of Dong Quai:

1. **Hormone Regulation:** Dong Quai contains phytoestrogens that mimic the effects of estrogen in the body, helping to balance hormone levels. This makes it particularly beneficial for women experiencing hormonal imbalances such as PMS, irregular periods, and menopausal symptoms.

2. **Pain Relief:** Dong Quai has anti-inflammatory properties that can help relieve menstrual cramps, joint pain, and headaches. It is also known for its mild analgesic effects.

3. **Blood Health:** Dong Quai is rich in iron and vitamin B12, which can help improve blood circulation and prevent anemia. It also contains coumarins, which have blood-thinning properties that may reduce the risk of blood clots.

4. **Immune Support:** Dong Quai has antioxidant properties that can help boost the immune system and protect the body from oxidative stress and inflammation.

5. **Digestive Health:** Dong Quai has been traditionally used to aid digestion and relieve symptoms of bloating, gas,

and indigestion.

Side Effects and Warnings:

While Dong Quai is generally well-tolerated by most people, there are some potential side effects and precautions to be aware of:

1. **Allergic Reactions:** Some people may be allergic to Dong Quai and experience symptoms such as rash, itching, or swelling. It is recommended to do a patch test before using Dong Quai topically or internally.

2. **Blood Thinning:** Because Dong Quai has blood-thinning properties, individuals taking blood thinners or with bleeding disorders should consult with their healthcare provider before using Dong Quai to avoid potential interactions.

3. **Pregnancy and Breastfeeding:** Dong Quai may stimulate uterine contractions and should be avoided by pregnant women to prevent miscarriage. It is also not recommended for breastfeeding mothers as it can pass through breast milk.

Recommended Dosages:

The appropriate dosage of Dong Quai can vary depending on the individual's age, health condition, and intended use. It is typically available in various forms such as capsules, tinctures, teas, and dried root powder.

Here are some general dosage guidelines:

1. **Capsules:** The typical dosage for Dong Quai capsules is 500-1000 mg per day, divided into two or more doses.

2. **Tincture:** For Dong Quai tinctures, the recommended dosage is 1-2 ml, diluted in water, up to three times per day.

3. **Tea:** To make Dong Quai tea, steep 1-2 teaspoons of dried root in hot water for 10-15 minutes. Drink up to three cups per day.

It is always best to consult with a qualified healthcare provider before starting any new herbal supplement, especially if you have any pre-existing health conditions or are taking medications. They can provide personalized recommendations and ensure that Dong Quai is safe and appropriate for your individual needs.

Fenugreek Seeds

Fenugreek seeds, also known as methi seeds, are a popular herb used in Indian cuisine for their distinctive flavor and numerous health benefits. These small, amber-colored seeds have been used for centuries in traditional medicine to treat a variety of ailments, making them a valuable addition to any kitchen or medicine cabinet.

Benefits of Fenugreek Seeds:

1. **Digestive Health:** Fenugreek seeds are rich in fiber, which helps to promote healthy digestion and prevent constipation. They also have natural anti-inflammatory properties that can help soothe an upset stomach.

2. **Blood Sugar Control:** Studies have shown that fenugreek seeds may help to lower blood sugar levels in people with diabetes, making them a valuable supplement for managing this chronic condition.

3. **Breast Milk Production:** Nursing mothers often use fenugreek seeds to help increase milk production and promote lactation. The seeds are believed to stimulate the production of prolactin, a hormone that plays a key role in milk production.

4. **Weight Management:** Fenugreek seeds have been shown to help regulate appetite and promote weight loss. The fiber in the seeds helps to keep you feeling full for longer, reducing the urge to overeat.

5. **Anti-inflammatory Properties:** Fenugreek seeds contain compounds that have been shown to have anti-inflammatory effects, making them useful

for managing conditions like arthritis and other inflammatory diseases.

Side Effects and Warnings:

While fenugreek seeds are generally safe for most people when consumed in moderate amounts, they can cause some side effects in certain individuals. These may include:

1. **Allergic Reactions:** Some people may be allergic to fenugreek seeds and can experience symptoms like itching, swelling, or difficulty breathing after consuming them.

2. **Blood Sugar Imbalance:** If you have diabetes or are taking medications to regulate blood sugar levels, it's important to monitor your blood sugar closely when consuming fenugreek seeds, as they may cause fluctuations in glucose levels.

3. **Digestive Issues:** In some cases, fenugreek seeds can cause gastrointestinal symptoms like gas, bloating, or diarrhea, especially if consumed in large quantities.

4. **Pregnant Women:** Pregnant women should avoid consuming fenugreek seeds in large amounts, as they may stimulate uterine contractions and potentially lead to premature labor.

Recommended Dosages:

The recommended dosage of fenugreek seeds can vary depending on the intended use. For general health benefits, most experts recommend consuming 1-2 teaspoons of fenugreek seeds daily, either whole or ground. For specific purposes like increasing milk production in nursing mothers, higher doses may be needed, but it's important to consult with a healthcare provider before exceeding recommended dosages.

Lastly, fenugreek seeds are a versatile herb with a range of health benefits, from promoting digestive health to controlling blood sugar levels. While they are generally safe for most people when consumed in moderation, it's important to be aware of potential side effects and consult with a healthcare provider before incorporating them into your diet or supplement regimen. With the right precautions, fenugreek seeds can be a valuable addition to your wellness routine.

Lemon Juice

Lemon juice is a popular natural remedy that has been used for centuries for its numerous health benefits. From weight loss to improved digestion, lemon juice is a versatile ingredient that can be easily incorporated into your daily routine. Let's explore the benefits, side effects, warnings, and recommended dosages of lemon juice.

Benefits:

1. **Weight loss:** Lemon juice is a great addition to a weight loss regimen as it helps to boost metabolism and aid digestion. The citric acid in lemon juice helps to break down fats and carbohydrates, making it easier for the body to process and eliminate them.

2. **Improved digestion:** Lemon juice is known to stimulate the production of digestive enzymes, which can help to improve digestion and prevent digestive issues such as bloating and constipation.

3. **Immune system support:** Lemon juice is rich in vitamin C, which is essential for a healthy immune system. Vitamin C helps to boost the production of white blood cells, which are responsible for fighting off infections and illnesses.

4. **Skin health:** The antioxidants in lemon juice can help to reduce inflammation and protect the skin from damage caused by free radicals. Drinking lemon juice regularly can help to improve the appearance of the skin and promote a healthy, glowing complexion.

Side effects:

While lemon juice is generally considered safe for most people, there are some potential side effects to be aware of. Some people may experience heartburn or acid reflux when consuming lemon juice, especially if they have a sensitive stomach. In rare cases, excessive consumption of lemon juice can lead to tooth erosion due to its high acid content. It is important to drink lemon juice in moderation and to rinse your mouth with water after drinking it to protect your teeth.

Warnings:

If you have a sensitive stomach or a history of acid reflux, it is best to consult with a healthcare provider before incorporating lemon juice into your diet. Additionally, if you are taking any medications, especially those that can interact with citrus fruits, such as certain antibiotics or blood pressure medications, it is important to talk to your doctor before increasing your intake of lemon juice.

Recommended dosages:

To enjoy the benefits of lemon juice without experiencing any adverse effects, it is recommended to drink diluted lemon juice in water. Start by squeezing the juice of half a lemon into a glass of warm water and gradually increase the amount of lemon juice as tolerated. Aim to drink lemon water first thing in the morning on an empty stomach for optimal benefits.

Finally, lemon juice is a powerful natural remedy with numerous health benefits. By incorporating lemon juice into your daily routine in moderation, you can enjoy improved digestion, weight loss support, and immune system boost. Remember to consult with your healthcare provider before making any significant changes to your diet to ensure that lemon juice is safe for you.

Neem

Neem, also known as Azadirachta indica, is a tree native to the Indian subcontinent that has been used for centuries in traditional medicine. The neem tree is known for its bitter taste and strong aroma, which is why it is often referred to as the "wonder tree" or the "village pharmacy." Neem is known for its various health benefits, including its antibacterial, antifungal, and anti-inflammatory properties.

Benefits of Neem:

- Neem is commonly used to treat skin conditions such as acne, eczema, and psoriasis due to its antibacterial and anti-inflammatory properties.

- Neem is also believed to have antifungal properties, making it effective in treating fungal infections such as athlete's foot and ringworm.

- Neem has been used to promote oral health by reducing plaque, preventing cavities, and treating gum disease.

- Neem is believed to have antioxidant properties, which can help protect cells from damage caused by free radicals.

- Neem is also used as a natural insect repellent and pesticide, as it is toxic to many pests but safe for humans.

Side Effects of Neem:

While neem is generally considered safe when used in recommended doses, there are some potential side effects to be aware of. These may include:

- Allergic reactions in some individuals, particularly those with allergies to plants in the Asteraceae family.

- Upset stomach or diarrhea when consumed in large doses.

- Neem oil can cause skin irritation or allergic reactions in some individuals when applied topically.

Warnings:

- Pregnant or breastfeeding women should consult with a healthcare professional before using neem, as there is limited research on its safety during pregnancy or lactation.

- Individuals with pre-existing medical conditions or taking medications should also consult with a healthcare professional before using neem, as it may interact with certain medications.

Recommended Dosages:

- Neem is available in various forms, including capsules, powders, extracts, and oils. The recommended dosage of neem may vary depending on the form and intended use. It is important to follow the manufacturer's instructions or consult with a healthcare professional for guidance on dosage.

- When using neem oil topically, it is recommended to dilute it with a carrier oil such as coconut or almond oil to avoid skin irritation.

- For oral use, neem capsules or powders can be taken according to the manufacturer's recommendations.

Neem is a versatile plant with a wide range of health benefits when used appropriately. However, it is important to be aware of potential side effects, warnings, and recommended dosages to ensure safe and effective use. Consulting with a healthcare professional before using neem can help ensure its benefits are maximized while minimizing any risks.

Papaya Seeds

Papaya seeds, often overlooked as a byproduct of the delicious fruit, pack a powerful punch when it comes to health benefits. These tiny seeds are rich in nutrients and contain unique enzymes that can help improve digestion, cleanse the liver, and even protect against certain diseases. However, like any supplement, it is important to understand the potential side effects, warnings, and recommended dosages of papaya seeds.

Benefits of Papaya Seeds:

Papaya seeds are a rich source of antioxidants, which can help protect the body from free radical damage and reduce inflammation. These seeds also contain a unique enzyme called papain, which has been shown to aid in digestion by breaking down proteins and improving nutrient absorption.

Additionally, papaya seeds have been found to have antibacterial and antiviral properties, making them a great natural remedy for fighting off infections and boosting the immune system. They have also been shown to have anti-inflammatory effects, which can help reduce pain and swelling in the body.

Furthermore, papaya seeds are a good source of essential nutrients such as magnesium, potassium, and fiber, which can help support overall health and well-being.

There is limited scientific research on the use of papaya seeds as a form of birth control or contraceptive. However, there are some studies and anecdotal evidence that suggest that papaya seeds may have some contraceptive properties.

One study published in the Journal of Ethnopharmacology in 1995 found that papaya seeds had contraceptive effects in male rats when given orally at high doses. The researchers found that the rats had reduced fertility and lower sperm counts after consuming papaya seeds for a certain period of time.

In traditional medicine, papaya seeds have been used as a natural contraceptive by women in some cultures. It is believed that consuming papaya seeds in large quantities can reduce fertility and prevent pregnancy. However, the effectiveness and safety of this method have not been scientifically proven.

It is important to note that using papaya seeds as a form of birth control may not be safe or effective. More research is needed to determine the potential contraceptive properties of papaya seeds and their safety for human use. It is always recommended to consult with a healthcare provider before trying any natural or herbal remedies for contraception.

Side Effects of Papaya Seeds:

While papaya seeds offer numerous health benefits, it is important to be aware of potential side effects. Some individuals may experience digestive issues such as bloating, gas, or diarrhea when consuming papaya seeds, especially in large quantities.

Papaya seeds also contain compounds called benzyl isothiocyanate and papain, which can be toxic in high doses. Pregnant women should avoid consuming papaya seeds, as these compounds could potentially harm the developing fetus.

Warnings and Recommended Dosages:

It is recommended to start with a small amount of papaya seeds and gradually increase the dosage as needed. The recommended dosage of papaya seeds is typically around 1 teaspoon per day for adults, taken either whole or ground up and mixed with food or beverages.

Individuals with digestive conditions or allergies to papaya should consult with a healthcare provider before adding papaya seeds to their diet. It is also important to source organic, non-GMO papaya seeds to ensure the highest quality and purity.

So, papaya seeds offer a wide range of health benefits, from improving digestion to boosting the immune system. However, it is important to be mindful of potential side effects and to follow the recommended dosages to ensure safe and effective use. By incorporating papaya seeds into your diet in moderation, you can reap the many benefits that these powerful seeds have to offer.

Pennyroyal (Mentha pulegium)

Pennyroyal, also known as Mentha pulegium, is a perennial herb belonging to the mint family. It is native to Europe, North Africa, and Southwest Asia. Pennyroyal has been used for centuries as a medicinal herb due to its numerous health benefits. *However, it is important to note that the plant contains potent compounds that can be toxic if consumed in large amounts.* In this chapter, we will explore the benefits, side effects, warnings, and recommended dosages of pennyroyal.

Benefits:

Pennyroyal is commonly used for its digestive properties. It has been traditionally used to alleviate symptoms of indigestion, bloating, and gas. The herb is also known for its antispasmodic properties, which can help to relax the muscles of the digestive tract and ease stomach cramps.

Additionally, pennyroyal is often used as a natural insect repellent. Its strong scent can deter mosquitoes and other biting insects. Some people also use pennyroyal oil topically to soothe insect bites and relieve itching.

Pennyroyal has also been used historically as a menstrual aid. It is believed to help regulate menstrual cycles and relieve symptoms of PMS. However, it is important to note that pennyroyal should not be used by pregnant women as it can induce abortion.

Side Effects:

While pennyroyal can offer several health benefits, it is important to use it with caution. The plant contains pulegone, a compound that can be toxic in large doses. Ingesting pennyroyal oil or large amounts of the herb can lead to serious side effects such as liver damage, kidney failure, and even death.

Ingesting pennyroyal can also cause symptoms such as nausea, vomiting, abdominal pain, dizziness, and confusion. In severe cases, it can lead to seizures and respiratory failure. It is crucial to seek medical attention immediately if you experience any of these symptoms after ingesting pennyroyal.

Warnings:

Pennyroyal should not be used by pregnant women, as it can cause uterine contractions and potentially lead to miscarriage. It should also be avoided by breastfeeding women, as the compounds in the herb can be passed to the infant through breast milk.

Individuals with liver or kidney problems should also avoid using pennyroyal, as it can exacerbate these conditions. Those with allergies to plants in the mint family (such as peppermint or spearmint) may also experience allergic reactions to pennyroyal.

Recommended Dosages:

Due to the potential toxicity of pennyroyal, it is important to use it in moderation. The recommended dosage of pennyroyal tea is 1-2 teaspoons of dried herb steeped in a cup of hot water for 10-15 minutes. It is best to consume no more than two cups of pennyroyal tea per day.

Pennyroyal oil should never be ingested, as it is highly concentrated and can be toxic. Instead, it can be diluted in a carrier oil and used topically in small amounts to repel insects or relieve insect bites.

Pennyroyal can offer several health benefits when used properly and in moderation. However, it is important to be aware of the potential side effects and risks associated with this herb. Always consult with a healthcare provider before incorporating pennyroyal into your wellness routine.

Queen Anne's Lace (Daucus carota)

Queen Anne's Lace, also known as Daucus carota, is a beautiful flowering plant that is commonly found throughout North America, Europe, and Asia. It is a member of the Apiaceae family, which also includes parsley, dill, and fennel. Queen Anne's Lace is most recognized for its delicate white flowers that resemble lace, hence its name. However, what many people may not know is that this plant has a long history of medicinal uses dating back to ancient times.

Benefits of Queen Anne's Lace:

- Queen Anne's Lace has traditionally been used to treat a variety of ailments, including digestive issues, respiratory problems, and menstrual irregularities.

- The roots of the plant have diuretic properties, which can help to eliminate excess water and toxins from the body.

- Queen Anne's Lace is also believed to have antispasmodic and anti-inflammatory properties, making it beneficial for easing muscle cramps and reducing inflammation.

- Some studies suggest that Queen Anne's Lace may have antimicrobial properties, which could help to fight off infections and support overall immune health.

Side Effects of Queen Anne's Lace:

- While Queen Anne's Lace is generally considered safe for most people when taken in moderation, there are some potential side effects to be aware of.

- Allergic reactions may occur in some individuals, particularly those who are sensitive to plants in the Apiaceae family.

- Pregnant and breastfeeding women are advised to avoid using Queen Anne's Lace, as it may have uterine-stimulating effects that could potentially harm the fetus or newborn.

- In large amounts, Queen Anne's Lace can cause photosensitivity, making the skin more susceptible to sunburn. It is important to use sunscreen and avoid prolonged sun exposure when taking this herb.

Warnings and Precautions:

- It is important to consult a healthcare provider before using Queen Anne's Lace, especially if you are pregnant, breastfeeding, or have any underlying health conditions.

- Queen Anne's Lace should not be used as a substitute for prescribed medications or medical treatments.

- Do not consume Queen Anne's Lace if you are allergic to plants in the Apiaceae family, such as carrots, parsley, or celery.

- Always follow recommended dosages and instructions when using Queen Anne's Lace to minimize the risk of side effects.

Recommended Dosages:

- Queen Anne's Lace can be taken in several forms, including as a tea, tincture, or capsule.

- For digestive issues and bloating, a cup of Queen Anne's Lace tea made from 1-2 teaspoons of dried herb steeped in boiling water for 10-15 minutes can be beneficial.

- Tinctures can be taken in doses of 1-2 milliliters up to three times per day, diluted in water or juice.

- Capsules containing Queen Anne's Lace extract are

also available, with recommended dosages varying depending on the specific product.

Queen Anne's Lace is a versatile herb with a range of potential health benefits. However, it is essential to use caution and consult with a healthcare provider before incorporating this herb into your wellness routine. By following recommended dosages and precautions, you can safely enjoy the therapeutic properties of Queen Anne's Lace.

Red Clover

The Red Clover, scientifically known as Trifolium pratense, is a perennial flowering plant that belongs to the legume family. It has been used for centuries in traditional medicine for its numerous health benefits. Let's explore the benefits, side effects, warnings, and recommended dosages of red clover.

Benefits of Red Clover:

1. **Hormone balance:** Red clover contains isoflavones, which are phytoestrogens that mimic the effects of estrogen in the body. This can help to alleviate symptoms of menopause, such as hot flashes, night sweats, and mood swings.

2. **Cardiovascular health:** Studies have shown that red clover may help to lower cholesterol levels and reduce the risk of heart disease. It also has anti-inflammatory properties that can help to protect the heart and blood vessels.

3. **Anti-cancer effects:** Some research suggests that the isoflavones in red clover may have anti-cancer properties, particularly in preventing breast and prostate cancers. However, more studies are needed to confirm these findings.

4. **Skin health:** Red clover has been used topically to treat skin conditions such as eczema and psoriasis. It is believed to have anti-inflammatory and antibacterial properties that can help to soothe irritated skin.

Side Effects of Red Clover:

While red clover is generally considered safe for most people when taken in moderate amounts, there are some potential side effects to be aware of. These may include:

1. **Allergic reactions:** Some individuals may experience allergic reactions to red clover, such as itching, rash, or swelling. If you have a known allergy to legumes, you should avoid using red clover.

2. **Hormonal effects:** Because red clover contains phytoestrogens, it may have hormonal effects on the body. Women who are pregnant, breastfeeding, or have a history of hormone-sensitive conditions should consult with their healthcare provider before using red clover.

3. **Bleeding disorders:** Red clover may have a blood-thinning effect, so individuals with bleeding disorders or those taking blood-thinning medications should use caution when using red clover.

Warnings and Precautions:

Before using red clover, it is important to consult with a healthcare provider, especially if you have any underlying health conditions or are taking medications. Additionally, consider the following precautions:

1. **Avoid long-term use:** While short-term use of red clover is generally safe, there is limited information on the long-term safety of this herb. It is recommended to use red clover for no more than 6-12 months at a time.

2. **Consult with a healthcare provider:** If you are pregnant, breastfeeding, have a hormone-sensitive condition, or are taking medications, it is important to consult with a healthcare provider before using red clover.

Recommended Dosages:

The dosages for red clover can vary depending on the form of the herb (capsules, tea, tincture) and the specific health condition being treated. However, the following dosages are commonly recommended:

1. **Dried herb:** 1-2 teaspoons of dried red clover flowers steeped in hot water for 10-15 minutes to make a tea, consumed 2-3 times per day.

2. **Capsules:** Follow the dosage instructions on the product label. Typically, 40-160mg of red clover extract is taken 1-2 times per day.

3. **Tincture:** Follow the dosage instructions on the product label. Typically, 1-2mL of red clover tincture is taken 2-3 times per day.

Red clover is a versatile and beneficial herb that can be used to support hormone balance, cardiovascular health, and skin health. While it is generally safe for most people, it is important to use caution, consult with a healthcare provider, and follow recommended dosages when using red clover.

Red Raspberry Leaf

Red raspberry leaf, also known as Rubus idaeus, has been used for centuries as a natural remedy for various health conditions. This herb is widely known for its many health benefits and is commonly used to promote women's health, particularly during pregnancy and childbirth. Let's explore the benefits, side effects, warnings, and recommended dosages of red raspberry leaf.

Benefits:

Red raspberry leaf is packed with nutrients and antioxidants that can benefit overall health. Some of the key benefits of red raspberry leaf include:

1. **Women's Health:** Red raspberry leaf is commonly used by women to enhance fertility, regulate menstrual cycles, and support a healthy pregnancy. This herb is known to strengthen and tone the uterus, which can help to facilitate easier labor and reduce the risk of complications during childbirth.

2. **Digestive Health:** Red raspberry leaf is also believed to support digestive health by reducing inflammation in the gastrointestinal tract and promoting healthy digestion. It can help to alleviate symptoms of indigestion, bloating, and constipation.

3. **Anti-Inflammatory Properties:** Red raspberry leaf contains anti-inflammatory compounds that can help to reduce inflammation and pain in the body. This makes it a popular remedy for conditions such as arthritis, gout, and muscle soreness.

4. **Immune Support:** The antioxidants in red raspberry leaf

can help to strengthen the immune system and protect the body from various infections and illnesses. Regular consumption of this herb may help to prevent colds, flu, and other common infections.

Side Effects:

While red raspberry leaf is generally considered safe for most people, it may cause some side effects in certain individuals. Some potential side effects of red raspberry leaf include:

1. Mild gastrointestinal upset, such as stomach cramps, nausea, and diarrhea.

2. Allergic reactions, such as rash, itching, and swelling.

3. Hormonal effects, such as changes in menstrual flow or duration.

If you experience any negative side effects after taking red raspberry leaf, it is recommended to discontinue use and consult with a healthcare provider.

Warnings:

Before using red raspberry leaf, it is important to consider the following warnings:

1. **Pregnancy:** While red raspberry leaf is commonly used to support pregnancy, it is important to consult with a healthcare provider before using this herb during pregnancy. Some studies suggest that red raspberry leaf may help to shorten labor and reduce the risk of complications, but more research is needed to confirm these benefits.

2. **Allergies:** If you have allergies to other plants in the Rubus genus, such as blackberry or strawberry, you may also be allergic to red raspberry leaf. It is important to test for allergies before using this herb.

3. **Medication Interactions:** Red raspberry leaf may interact with certain medications, especially blood-

thinning medications and hormone therapies. It is important to consult with a healthcare provider before using this herb if you are taking any medications.

Recommended Dosages:

The recommended dosage of red raspberry leaf may vary depending on the form of the herb and the individual's health needs. In general, the following dosages are commonly recommended:

1. **Tea:** To make red raspberry leaf tea, steep 1-2 teaspoons of dried herb in hot water for 10-15 minutes. Drink 1-3 cups of tea per day.

2. **Capsules:** Take 1-2 capsules of red raspberry leaf supplement per day, following the manufacturer's instructions.

3. **Tincture:** Take 1-2 dropperfuls of red raspberry leaf tincture in water or juice, up to three times per day.

It is important to start with a low dose of red raspberry leaf and gradually increase the dosage as needed. It is also recommended to consult with a healthcare provider before using red raspberry leaf to determine the appropriate dosage for your individual needs.

Red raspberry leaf is a valuable herb with numerous health benefits, particularly for women's health. While it is generally safe for most people, it is important to be aware of potential side effects, warnings, and recommended dosages before using this herb. By following these guidelines and consulting with a healthcare provider, you can safely incorporate red raspberry leaf into your wellness routine and enjoy its many health benefits.

Tansy

Tansy, a perennial herb native to Europe and Asia, has been used for centuries for its medicinal properties. It is known for its bright yellow flowers and distinctive aroma. In this chapter, we will discuss the benefits, side effects, warnings, and recommended dosages of tansy.

Benefits of Tansy:

1. **Digestive Aid:** Tansy is often used to aid digestion and relieve symptoms of bloating, gas, and indigestion.

2. **Menstrual Relief:** Tansy has been traditionally used to alleviate menstrual cramps and regulate menstrual cycles.

3. **Anti-inflammatory:** Tansy contains compounds that have anti-inflammatory properties, making it useful for treating conditions such as arthritis and joint pain.

4. **Antimicrobial:** Tansy has antimicrobial properties that can help fight off infections and boost the immune system.

5. **Skin Health:** Tansy can be used topically to soothe skin conditions such as eczema, psoriasis, and acne.

Side Effects of Tansy:

1. **Allergic Reactions:** Some individuals may be allergic to tansy, resulting in symptoms such as hives, itching, and swelling.

2. **Liver Toxicity:** Tansy contains compounds that can be toxic to the liver if consumed in large quantities or for an extended period of time.

3. **Pregnant Women:** Pregnant women should avoid tansy as it may cause uterine contractions and possible miscarriage.

4. **Children and Pets:** Tansy should not be used on children or pets as it can be toxic if ingested.

Warnings:

1. Always consult with a healthcare professional before adding tansy to your regimen, especially if you have a medical condition or are taking medications.

2. Do not exceed the recommended dosage of tansy as it can be toxic in large amounts.

3. Purchase tansy from reputable sources to ensure its purity and quality.

Recommended Dosages:

1. The recommended dosage of tansy is typically 1-2 grams of dried herb per day, taken in capsule or tea form.

2. Tansy essential oil should be diluted before applying to the skin, as it can cause irritation in its concentrated form.

3. It is important to follow the instructions provided on tansy products or consult with a healthcare professional for personalized dosages.

Tansy has many health benefits but should be used with caution due to its potential side effects and toxicity. It is always best to consult with a healthcare professional before incorporating tansy into your wellness routine.

Tea Tree Oil

Tea tree oil, also known as melaleuca oil, is derived from the leaves of the tea tree plant (Melaleuca alternifolia). Native to Australia, tea tree oil has been used for centuries by indigenous Australians for its medicinal properties. Today, it is widely used in various skincare products, household cleaners, and aromatherapy.

Benefits of Tea Tree Oil

Tea tree oil is known for its antibacterial, antifungal, and anti-inflammatory properties. As a natural remedy, it has been used to treat a variety of skin conditions, including acne, athlete's foot, and eczema. It can also help alleviate symptoms of dandruff, insect bites, and minor cuts and scrapes.

In addition to its skin benefits, tea tree oil is also used for its antimicrobial properties. It can help disinfect wounds, clean surfaces, and even repel insects. Some studies have also suggested that tea tree oil may have antiviral properties, making it a potential treatment for cold sores and other viral infections.

Side Effects of Tea Tree Oil

While tea tree oil is generally considered safe when used topically, some individuals may experience skin irritation or allergic reactions. It is important to perform a patch test before using tea tree oil on a larger area of skin to determine if you are sensitive to it. In rare cases, tea tree oil can cause severe allergic reactions and should be avoided by anyone with a known allergy to the plant.

Ingesting tea tree oil is not recommended, as it can be toxic when taken orally. Swallowing even small amounts of tea tree oil can lead to symptoms such as nausea, vomiting, and diarrhea. If ingested in larger quantities, tea tree oil can cause more serious side effects, such as confusion, loss of consciousness, and coma. It is essential to keep tea tree oil out of the reach of children and pets to prevent accidental ingestion.

Warnings and Precautions

Pregnant or nursing women should exercise caution when using tea tree oil, as its safety during pregnancy and breastfeeding has not been established. It is always best to consult with a healthcare provider before using tea tree oil if you are pregnant or nursing.

Tea tree oil should also be used with caution on sensitive skin or areas of broken skin, as it may cause irritation or stinging. It is important to dilute tea tree oil with a carrier oil, such as coconut or olive oil, before applying it to the skin to minimize the risk of irritation.

Recommended Dosages

When using tea tree oil topically, it is recommended to mix it with a carrier oil in a ratio of 1 to 10 (1 drop of tea tree oil to 10 drops of carrier oil). This will help prevent skin irritation and ensure proper absorption of the oil.

For acne treatment, apply a small amount of diluted tea tree oil to the affected area twice daily. For fungal infections, such as athlete's foot, apply diluted tea tree oil to the affected area and leave it on for several hours before rinsing off. It is essential to monitor your skin's reaction to tea tree oil and discontinue use if irritation occurs.

Tea tree oil offers a natural and versatile remedy for various skin conditions and minor ailments. By understanding its benefits, side effects, and proper usage, you can safely incorporate tea tree oil into your skincare routine and household cleaning

Wild Yam (Dioscorea villosa)

Wild yam, also known as Dioscorea villosa, is a perennial plant native to North America. It has been used for centuries by indigenous peoples for its medicinal properties and is now commonly used as a natural remedy for a variety of ailments. The root of the wild yam plant is the part that is typically used for medicinal purposes, and it can be consumed in various forms including capsules, tinctures, or teas.

Benefits of Wild Yam:

Wild yam is believed to have several health benefits, including:

- **Hormonal balance:** Wild yam contains diosgenin, a compound that is structurally similar to progesterone. As a result, wild yam is often used to help balance hormones in women, especially during menopause or menstruation.

- **Menstrual cramps:** Wild yam is believed to have antispasmodic properties, making it beneficial for relieving menstrual cramps and other menstrual symptoms.

- **Digestive health:** Wild yam is also thought to have mild anti-inflammatory properties, making it potentially beneficial for digestive issues such as irritable bowel syndrome (IBS) or gas and bloating.

- **Muscle and joint pain:** Some people use wild yam topically as a salve or cream to help alleviate muscle and joint pain.

Side Effects and Warnings:

While wild yam is generally considered safe for most people when taken in recommended doses, there are some potential side effects and warnings to be aware of:

- **Allergic reactions:** Some individuals may be allergic to wild yam, particularly those who are allergic to other plants in the yam family.

- **Interactions with medications:** Wild yam may interact with certain medications, such as blood thinners or hormonal contraceptives. It is always best to consult with a healthcare provider before taking wild yam, especially if you are taking any other medications.

- **Pregnancy and breastfeeding:** Pregnant or breastfeeding women should avoid taking wild yam, as it may have hormone-like effects that could affect pregnancy or breastfeeding.

Recommended Dosages:

The appropriate dosage of wild yam can vary depending on the form it is taken in, as well as the individual's age, weight, and health status. It is always best to follow the dosing instructions on the product label, or to consult with a healthcare provider to determine the appropriate dosage for your specific needs.

In general, the typical recommended dosage ranges from 2-6 grams of wild yam root per day, divided into two or three doses. It is important to start with a lower dose and gradually increase as needed to determine the most effective dosage for your individual needs.

Wild yam is a natural remedy with several potential health benefits, particularly for hormonal balance and menstrual issues. While it is generally considered safe for most people when taken in recommended doses, it is important to be aware of any potential side effects or interactions with medications. As with any herbal supplement, it is always best to consult with a healthcare provider before starting a new regimen.

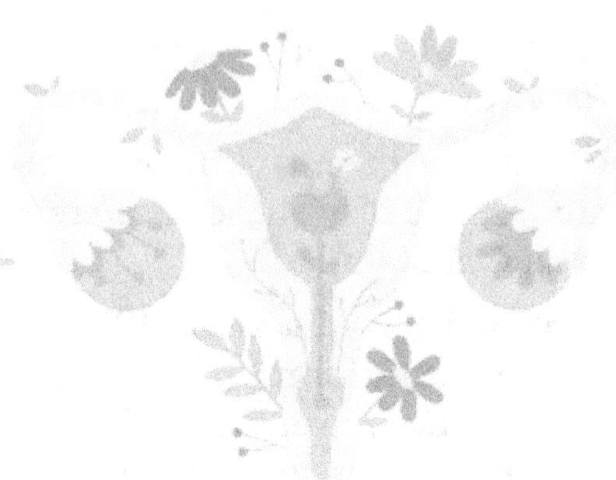

Resources

1. Mountain Rose Herbs Address: 4020 Stewart Road,Eugene, OR 97405 Phone Number: 800-879-3337 Website: www.mountainroseherbs.com

2. Starwest Botanicals Address: 161 Main Avenue, Sacramento, CA 95838 Phone Number: 800-800-4372 Website: www.starwest-botanicals.com

3. Herb Pharm Address: 101 Dry Creek Road, Williams, OR 97544 Phone Number: 800-348-4372 Website: www.herb-pharm.com

4. Gaia Herbs Address: 101 Gaia Herbs Drive, Brevard, NC 28712 Phone Number: 800-831-7780 Website: www.gaiaherbs.com

5. Frontier Co-op Address: 3021 78th Street, Norway, IA 52318 Phone Number: 800-669-3275 Website: www.frontiercoop.com

6. Nature's Sunshine Address: 2500 West Executive Parkway, Suite 500, Lehi, UT 84043 Phone Number: 800-223-8225 Website: www.naturessunshine.com

7. Pacific Botanicals Address: 4350 Fisherman Road, Grants Pass, OR 97526 Phone Number: 541-479-7777 Website: www.pacificbotanicals.com

8. Mountain Maus Remedies Address: 90 S. Alaska Street, Suite 101, Palmer, AK 99645 Phone Number: 907-745-5639 Website: www.alaskanessences.com

9. Blessed Herbs Address: 3775 Azurite Street, Riverside, CA 92509 Phone Number: 800-489-4372 Website: www.blessedherbs.com

10. The Herbalist Address: 2106 NE 65th Street, Seattle, WA 98115 Phone Number: 206-523-2600 Website: www.theherbalist.com

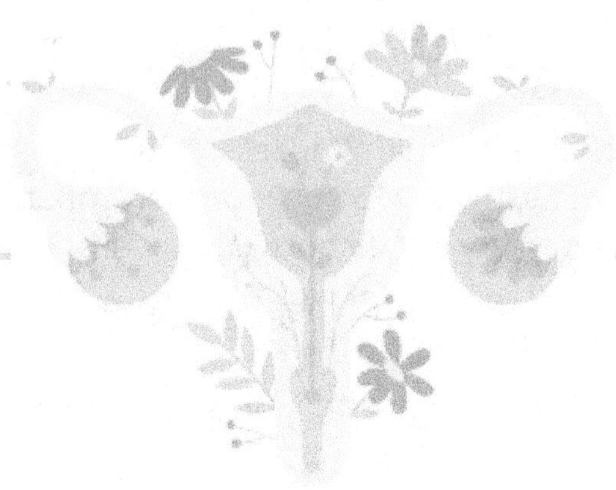

Herbal Medicine Books

1. "The Herbal Medicine-Maker's Handbook: A Home Manual" by James Green, Link: https://www.amazon.com/Herbal-Medicine-Makers-Handbook-Home/dp/0895949903
2. "The Encyclopedia of Natural Medicine" by Michael Murray and Joseph Pizzorno, Link: https://www.amazon.com/Encyclopedia-Natural-Medicine-Third-Bestselling/dp/1451663005
3. "Rosemary Gladstar's Herbal Recipes for Vibrant Health: 175 Teas, Tonics, Oils, Salves, Tinctures, and Other Natural Remedies for the Entire Family" by Rosemary Gladstar, Link: https://www.amazon.com/Rosemary-Gladstars-Herbal-Recipes-Vibrant/dp/1603420789
4. "Rodale's 21st-Century Herbal: A Practical Guide for Healthy Living Using Nature's Most Powerful Plants" by Michael Balick, Link: https://www.amazon.com/Rodales-21st-Century-Herbal-21st-Century/

dp/1609614571

5. "The Complete Herbal Guide: A Natural Approach to Healing" by Stacey Chillemi, Link: https://www.amazon.com/Complete-Herbal-Guide-Natural-Approach/dp/0984384955

6. "The Modern Herbal Dispensatory: A Medicine-Making Guide" by Thomas Easley and Steven Horne, Link: https://www.amazon.com/Modern-Herbal-Dispensatory-Medicine-Making-Guide/dp/1623170794

7. "Healing Herbal Teas: Learn to Blend 101 Specially Formulated Teas for Stress Management, Common Ailments, Seasonal Health, and Immune Support" by Sarah Farr, Link: https://www.amazon.com/Healing-Herbal-Teas-Management-Support/dp/161212995X

8. "The Way of Herbs: Fully Updated with the Latest Developments in Herbal Science" by Michael Tierra, Link: https://www.amazon.com/Way-Herbs-Updated-Developments-Herbal/dp/0671023276

9. "The One Earth Herbal Sourcebook: Everything You Need to Know About Chinese, Western, and Ayurvedic Herbal Treatments", by Alan Keith Tillotson Ph.D. (Author), Nai-shing Hu Tillotson O.M.D. (Contributor), Robert Abel (Contributor), Link: https://www.amazon.com/One-Earth-Herbal-Sourcebook-Everything/dp/1575666170

10. "The Herbal Apothecary: 100 Medicinal Herbs and How to Use Them", Dr. JJ Pursell (Author), https://www.amazon.com/Herbal-Apothecary-Medicinal-Herbs-Them/dp/1604695676

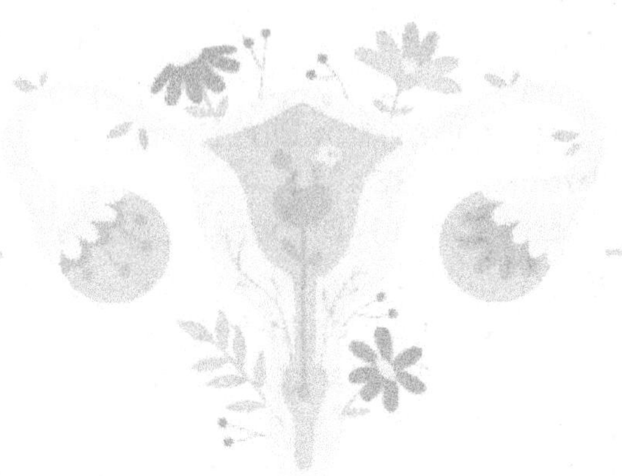

Research Papers

1. "Herbal contraceptives: Exploring the mechanisms of action" - https://www.researchgate.net/publication/322595515_Herbal_contraceptives_Exploring_the_mechanisms_of_action

2. "Herbal birth control methods: A review" - https://pubmed.ncbi.nlm.nih.gov/32347167/

3. "Efficacy of herbal medicines in birth control: A systematic review" - https://journals.sagepub.com/doi/abs/10.1177/2156587218818680

4. "Herbal contraception: An alternative approach" - https://www.tandfonline.com/doi/full/10.3109/19390211.2013.782960

5. "Herbal contraceptives: A review of their efficacy and safety" - https://www.researchgate.net/publication/315076934_Herbal_contraceptives_A_revi

ew_of_their_efficacy_and_safety

6. "The use of herbal contraceptives among women in rural areas: A qualitative study" - https://bmccomplementmedtherapies.biomedcentral.com/articles/10.1186/s12906-019-2490-3

7. "Herbal birth control: A literature review" - https://www.researchgate.net/publication/220236655_Herbal_birth_control_A_literature_review

8. "The potential of herbal contraceptives in family planning: A review" - https://www.tandfonline.com/doi/abs/10.1080/09712119.2010.10506169

9. "Herbal contraception: A systematic review of traditional practices and scientific evidence" - https://doi.org/10.1089/acm.2008.0443

10. "Herbal methods of family planning among women in rural India: A cross-sectional study" - https://www.ncbi.nlm.nih.gov/pmc/articles/PMC5111701/

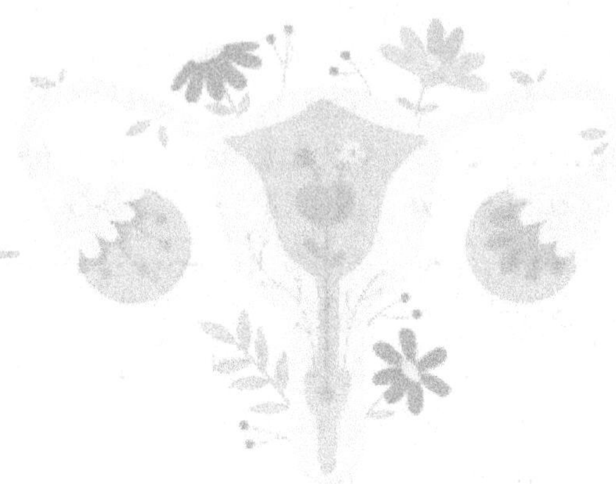

References

1. "Herbal Birth Control" by Aviva Romm (book)

2. "Herbal Contraception" by Deb Soule (book)

3. "Wild Feminine: Finding Power, Spirit & Joy in the Female Body" by Tami Kent (book)

4. "Garden of Fertility: A Guide to Charting Your Fertility Signals to Prevent or Achieve Pregnancy-Naturally-and to Gauge Your Reproductive Health" by Katie Singer (book)

5. "The Complete Book of Herbs for Natural Health" by Penelope Ody (book)

6. "The Birth Control Revolution" by Janet Golden (book)

7. "Herbal Contraception and Abortion: A Comprehensive Study of the Practice of the Nineteenth Century" by Colette Praeger (book)

8. "Herbal Medicine for Women: How to use herbs in a

woman's natural healing journey" by Marija Helt (book)

9. "Red Moon Passage: The Power and Wisdom of Menstruation" by Bonnie J. Horrigan (book)

10. "The Wild Genie: The Healing Power of Menstruation" by Alexandra Pope (book)

11. "WomanCode: Perfect Your Cycle, Amplify Your Fertility, Supercharge Your Sex Drive, and Become a Power Source" by Alisa Vitti (book)

12. "The Fertile Female: How the Power of Longing for a Child Can Save Your Life and Change the World" by Julia Indichova (book)

13. "The Woman's Herbal Apothecary: 200 Natural Remedies for Healing, Hormone Balance, Beauty and Longevity, and Creating Calm" by J. J. Pursell (book)

14. Herbal Birth Control - http://www.positivehealth.com/article/herbal-medicine/herbal-birth-control

15. Herbal Contraception for women - http://www.globalherbalsupplies.com/herbal-library/herbal-contraception/

16. Herbal Contraceptive Methods - http://www.nyrp.org.uk/meth_herbal.html

17. Natural Herbal Contraception for Women - http://www.yourtango.com/2014207119/herbal-contraceptive-options

18. Herbal Contraception: A Review of the Research - http://www.learn.pharmacy.unc.edu/herbalcontraception/

19. Herbal Contraception and Abortion and Herbal Codical and Abrotatifaction: A Female Task Performed by Women - http://www.phillyvoice.com/herbal-contraception-and-abortion

20. Herbal Birth Control- http://www.positivehealth.com/

article/herbal-medicine/herbal-birth-control

21. Traditional Herbal Contraception and Family Planning - http://www.who.int/bulletin/volumes/88/2/09-085993/en/

22. Herbal Contraception - http://www.academia.edu/1783024/Herbal_Contraception

23. Herbs for Life: Herbal Contraception - http://www.all-natural.com/herbcom6.html

24. Naturopathic Medicine: Herbal Birth Control - http://www.pacificcollege.edu/news/blog/2015/02/28/naturopathic-medicine-herbal-birth-control

25. Herbal Contraception - http://www.researchgate.net/publication/257690577_Herbal_Contraception

About The Author

Kimberly Hodge, Lmt, Nhc, Chn

As a retired career college instructor in the wellness field, Kimberly has a vast amount of knowledge in health and wellness topics as a Natural Health Consultant, Certified in Holistic Nutrition, and a Licensed Massage Therapist. In addition, she also has many years of experience owning and operating several successful small businesses. She 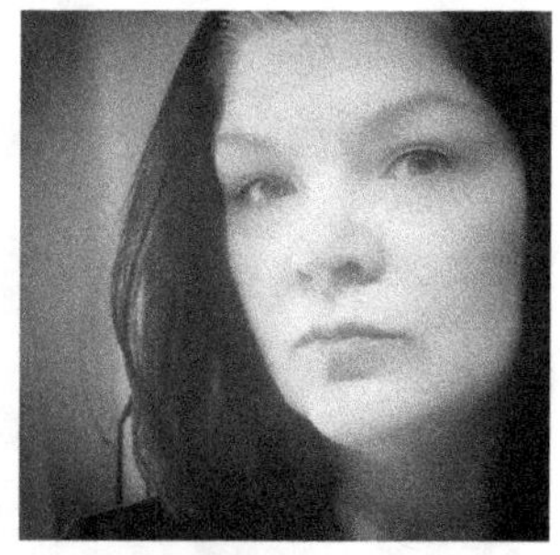 now focuses on her writing. She enjoys writing in the health and wellness, business, and spiritual genre. When Kimberly is not writing she enjoys spending time with her husband and their fur baby.

Anxiety: Find Relief Naturally

"Find Peace from Anxiety Naturally and Transform Your Life"
We all suffer from anxiety from time to time in our lives, but for some of us, it can be a daily struggle. Anxiety can lead to a multitude of health issues including, sleep disturbances, increased blood pressure, irritability, extreme fatigue, relationship issues, and more - all leading to even more anxiety!

In this book, you will find personal experiences, quick tips, and healthy strategies to help calm the mind naturally. The strategies in this book you can use anytime to help promote calm and peace of mind. You will learn some of the common causes of anxiety, how to help yourself, and what to do when you think you need professional help.

And lastly, learn how changing your self-talk, using the law of attraction, simple breathing, and ground techniques can help you calm your anxiety quickly.

Overcoming Medical Trauma And Thriving

Medical trauma can stem from a wide range of experiences, such as surgery, serious illnesses, medical errors, invasive procedures, or hospitalizations. The impact of medical trauma can be significant and may manifest in various ways, including anxiety, depression, post-traumatic stress disorder (PTSD), and distrust of medical professionals.

It can also affect one's overall well-being, quality of life, and relationships. Understanding and acknowledging the impact of medical trauma is crucial in providing holistic and patient-centered care.

Key Topics Covered:

~Understanding Medical Trauma & Common Causes
~Identifying Personal Triggers & Coping Strategies
~Building Resilience and Self-Empowerment
~Seeking Professional Help and Support
~Alternative Healing and Modalities
~Moving Forward and Thriving

Whipple Surgery Survivor: One Woman's Journey With Pancreatic Intraductal Papillary Mucinous Neoplasms (Ipmn's)

Whipple Surgery Survivor – One Woman's Journey with Pancreatic Intraductal Papillary Mucinous Neoplasms (IPMN's), is one woman's personal journey having undergone the Whipple procedure – also known as the pancreaticoduodenectomy. This is a very complex surgery, commonly performed for pancreatic cancer patients.

Her personal journey going through the surgery, recovery, and the quality of life afterward, can be especially helpful for other patients, their caregivers, friends and family, and medical professionals. In this book, you will find helpful resources, how to prepare for the surgery, and what helped during her recovery.

Includes:

~How she prepared for surgery
~Day of Surgery
~Hospital Stay
~Recovery
~Complications
~Tips & Resources

Manifesting Happiness: A Practical Guide To Transforming Your Life

After reading this practical guide, you will find that you, too, can lead a life of happiness! Embrace the power within you to transform your existence into an exhilarating journey filled with joy and fulfillment. Unlock the secret sauce of happiness and let it permeate every aspect of your being, igniting a fire in your heart that burns brighter than ever before.

With each turn of the page, you'll discover invaluable tools and techniques that empower you to create a life that resonates with excitement and positivity. From fostering meaningful relationships to nurturing self-love, from pursuing passions relentlessly to finding gratitude in even the smallest moments - this guide unravels all the mysteries behind cultivating genuine happiness.

No longer will it be elusive or unattainable; instead, it will become a vibrant reality pulsating through your veins. The world is brimming with endless possibilities waiting for you to seize them; grab hold of life's adventure and savor every delicious moment on this thrilling path toward everlasting bliss!

www.ingramcontent.com/pod-product-compliance
Lightning Source LLC
Chambersburg PA
CBHW061052250726
48653CB00001B/370